The Effluent Eye

The Effluent Eye

Narratives for Decolonial Right-Making

Rosemary J. Jolly

University of Minnesota Press
Minneapolis
London

This book is freely available in an open access edition thanks to TOME (Toward an Open Monograph Ecosystem)—a collaboration of the Association of American Universities, the Association of University Presses, and the Association of Research Libraries—and the generous support of the Pennsylvania State University. Learn more at the TOME website: openmonographs.org.

Portions of the Preface, chapter 2, and chapter 5 were originally published as "Pandemic Crises: The Anthropocene as Pathogenic Cycle," *Interdisciplinary Studies in Literature and Environment* 27, no. 4 (2020): 809–22. Portions of the Introduction and chapter 1 are adapted from "Effluence, 'Waste,' and African Humanism: Extra-Anthropocentric Being and Human Rightness," *Social Dynamics* 44, no. 1 (2018): 158–78; copyright Taylor & Francis: https://www.tandfonline.com/doi/abs/10.1080/02533952.2018.1449723. Portions of the Introduction, chapter 2, chapter 3, and chapter 5 are adapted from "Decolonising 'Man,' Resituating Pandemic: An Intervention in the Pathogenesis of Colonial Capitalism," *Medical Humanities* 48, no. 2 (2022): 221–29; https://doi.org/10.1136/medhum-2021-012267.

Excerpts from Antjie Krog's "*Rondeau in Vier Diele*" and M. NourbeSe Philip's "Zong #1" are reprinted with permission of the authors.

Copyright 2023 by Rosemary J. Jolly

The Effluent Eye: Narratives for Decolonial Right-Making is licensed under a Creative Commons Attribution-NonCommercial 4.0 International License (CC BY-NC 4.0): creativecommons.org/licenses/by-nc/4.0/

Published by the University of Minnesota Press
111 Third Avenue South, Suite 290
Minneapolis, MN 55401–2520
http://www.upress.umn.edu

▰ Available as a Manifold edition at manifold.umn.edu

DOI: https://doi.org/10.5749/9781452970738
ISBN 978-1-5179-1568-1 (hc)
ISBN 978-1-5179-1569-8 (pb)

A Cataloging-in-Publication record for this book is available from the Library of Congress

The University of Minnesota is an equal-opportunity educator and employer.

UMP LSI

For my parents, Alan Jolly, Eve D'Aeth, Richard D'Aeth. Thank you for having me.

*And Chris McMullen,
who adopted the lands of my youth as his and therefore knows how to "get a robot," how the direction "drive until the small donga that comes after the big one" on the road to Massite can be difficult, how coffins can fall off bakkies on the road between Centocow and Ixopo, and what happens when you drink mampoer in the Groot-Marico on your way to the Kalahari.*

sonder godsdiens van buite
is hulle diere van binne
as diere het hulle geen siele van binne
van buite

sonder siele van binne
is hul gedoemdes van buite
is daar geen regte van binne
van diegene van buite
op land of op lewe
> —colonial view on Indigenous people, as described by Antije Krog in "Rondeau in vier Diele"

Contents

Positive Country: A Preface with Acknowledgments	xi
Introduction	1
1. Effluence, "Waste," and African Humanism: Extra-Anthropocentric Being and Human Right-Making	23
2. Effluence in Disease: Ebola and HIV as Case Studies of Debility in the Postcolonial State	49
3. Addiction and Its Formations under Capitalism: Refusing the Bubble and Effluent Persistence	87
4. Trauma "Exceptionalism" and Sexual Assault in Global Contexts: Methodologies and Epistemologies of the Effluent	123
5. Effluent Capacity and the Human Right-Making Artifact: Alexis Wright's *Carpentaria* as Geobiography	159
Afterword: Simultaneous Reading and Slow Becoming	183
Notes	193
Bibliography	205
Index	221

Positive Country

A Preface with Acknowledgments

I began writing this book in 2013, long before the outbreak of Covid-19 as a global pandemic in late 2019. I have lived through the AIDS pandemic and other epidemics—of tuberculosis, of typhoid, of cholera, of malaria. I had moved from working with the narratives of victim-survivors of state-sponsored torture to researching programs for prevention of gender-based violence (GBV) within HIV contexts. The issues were connected in that they both involved working with communities in contexts of extreme stigma, vulnerability, and resilience.[1]

The continuity between my work on narratives of state-sponsored torture and GBV prevention further developed my interest in violence in highly intersectional junctures of racially entangled colonial/postcolonial power differentials and gender inequities. Over the past two decades, it also became increasingly clear to me that the extremely capacious human rights written into the South African Constitution of 1994 were unable to protect most people from sexual abuse, and sometimes were even the cause of hostility (Jolly and Jeeves 2010).

The inequities I witnessed came home to roost in normative practices of Western medicine in ways that on occasion made Western medical interventions deleterious to those infected with and affected by HIV in rural South Africa. I have written about HIV in South Africa in the context of the transition from apartheid to a democracy and in my work on healthcare as a human right (Jolly and Jeeves 2010; Jolly 2010), but none of this had really touched on HIV as an environment, rather than an event, or the ways in which the pandemic's iteration in South Africa literally made me rethink death, not as an end but as a companion community to the living, not bound by human likeness, a concept I investigate in chapter 1.

In the protest days for free access to highly active antiretroviral therapy (HAART), in the urban areas, where stigma was not as great as in rural areas, the Treatment Action Campaign distributed T-shirts (maroon, if I remember correctly) with the slogan "HIV-positive" on them. The idea was to render "I am HIV-positive" unstigmatized, while simultaneously confusing spectators at rallies as to the actual identity of who was positive and who was not, because those of us supporting HIV-positive persons marched alongside them wearing HIV-positive T-shirts too, expressing our refusal to stigmatize HIV-positive persons and demanding that the government provide HAART. The creative fluidity of this move was the beginning of my thinking with effluence.

South Africa, including the countryside in a physical sense, was HIV-positive. Everywhere there was evidence of it: more freshly opened graves than old ones in a cemetery; water contaminated by bodies not buried properly owing to the prohibitive cost of burials for some; giant government-sponsored ads alongside roads sporting awareness messages; the forbidden subject exhibited everywhere in the physical environment; and the leaking of the disease into conversations about whether whites gave Blacks HIV in revenge for the 1994 election of Mandela and furtive conversations in bars about whether or not to test. In chapter 1, I go into the depth of mourning we experienced. Suffice it to say, for the moment, that effluence took on a new, personal, embodied meaning for me in the wake of my HIV work. HIV was effluent: it spread everywhere but was simultaneously too awful to be spoken about; its introduction into the spoken word required careful negotiation in discrete contexts. Yet it acted as Covid-19 is doing now, as an all-encompassing environment, despite attempts to name it as an event or discrete disease.

When I returned from sabbatical research in New Zealand by way of Melbourne in March 2020, in a rush to get back to the United States before the borders of Australia and Singapore closed, I was both horrified and engaged to witness the breakdown of what I call "the bubble," a phenomenon I investigate in some detail in chapter 3. I am not, I hope, filled with *schadenfreude,* but it was intriguing to see populations that usually think of themselves as protected struggling to find a way of being, a habitus, in this newly threatening environment. I was bewildered, critical, and enchanted by the array of responses, from a rush on toilet paper in Perth in the early days of the crisis to witnessing a young couple in Singapore airport in full (and I mean full) level-4 containment suits, strolling hand in hand through the duty-free section of the international departure area, in a flagrant display of commodified protection, a topic I revisit in chapter 2. In the business lounge (a business ticket was the only way to get back before the borders closed, and happily Penn State reimbursed me for that reason), families (though mostly men) involved in migrant labor in the global sense explained how they were being sent home, no matter how long their contracts were. Everyone was whispering into cell phones about how long each of them may have been exposed to the virus, what to tell the kids about why Dad was coming home early, and in between times, wiping cutlery and plates with alcohol-based sanitizer before plopping another set of snacks on a plate or cracking open a Perrier. When we got to Newark Liberty International, nothing had been sanitized . . . but also there was nobody there. To our chagrin, with all the shutdowns, we couldn't get coffee between Newark and State College, and so we drove to State College on empty, as it were, after the overnight flight. These were different signs of a "positive country" from those of South Africa I had experienced before, but I was clearly back in positive country.

In 2011, I was sitting around a campfire inside a boma,[2] at a comfortable but affordable game reserve on the Pongola River in the northernmost district of KwaZulu-Natal, South Africa. I found myself wondering about the isiZulu servants who made up our beds and kept us fed. We looked at the fauna and flora and had massages, while the servants, even if they were housed on the reserve, traversed the boundary between game sanctuary and impoverished surrounding areas to go about the business of living. At that time, the Pongola area, just south of the Swaziland border, had an HIV prevalence rate of 39.3 percent (South Africa National Department of Health 2012, 32). What, I wondered for the umpteenth time, did it mean to be driven around, mostly looking at megafauna, while these servants—who have an embodied intergenerational knowledge of white apprehensions of Blacks as baboons—were at our beck and call?[3] What kind of beings are animals, human and nonhuman, in positive country?

This nexus of humans, nonhuman wildlife, and disease has followed me all my life. I lived for three years as a child in the same medical residence as Steve Biko did: he was there at the same time. The Black medical residence, Alan Taylor, built as an army barracks in World War II in the ill-named Happy Valley, south of Durban, is now infamous for its pollution.[4] This sojourn preceded our move to the only mission hospital for thousands of square miles in the center of the independent kingdom of Lesotho. As a child, on the one hand, I had human companions who were never recognized as such at schools and other "White spaces" because they were amaZulu and Basotho, the generic "Blacks" of the apartheid era. On the other hand, I had nonhuman, animal companions: horses (the only way to get around in Lesotho, including to remote clinics), dogs, cats, and even Henry Bolognaise, a black-tailed kite who had a massive cage in our kitchen at Alan Taylor Residence, where he recovered from a broken wing and was then, finally, rehabilitated back into the wild by the Natal Parks Board of the day. (He was actually Basotho too, if birds have nationalities: he was brought to us by a herd-boy in the Mokhotlong district of eastern Lesotho when we were camping, and Dad splinted his broken wing with a kebab stick. We then smuggled him into South Africa via Sani Pass.) The nonhuman animals struck me as much more dependable in their interactions with humans than most humans around me as they interacted with each other.

I had a long way yet to go, however, before I could express the interdependence of us humans, nonhuman animals, and what we call our environment as I experience it. Even as I sat on a rock in Lesotho overlooking the King's grazing grounds as a thirteen-year-old, I knew the rock would be there long after I was gone, and I found that comforting. It would forever know I had sat there. I come back to the rock-as-witness in my final chapter. I couldn't have explained this to my family, who were legitimately busy curing people, and my classmates at boarding school in Bloemfontein would have thought I was utterly mad. Having an effluent eye can feel like being mad, without access to narrative concepts that make it make sense, as we shall see.

First, however, a note on methodology. Narrative is the primary subject matter on which I bring the effluent eye to bear. Fictional works and the histories of their contexts of production form these narratives, where relationships between narratives of history and those of fiction are seen as mutually constitutive through the making of genre. Viewing stories in conjunction with the histories of their genres is an excellent way to trace the entrenchment of colonialist-capitalist anthropocentrism, the context of human rights and its decolonial alternative, human right-making. The subjects of narrative discourse, fictional or nonfictional, are always in a radical sense invented: they manifest the discursive complicity of how we conceive ourselves semantically, and how we locate ourselves as subjects within discursive acts that themselves are co-constitutive of material and extramaterial frameworks.

A common way to render authority in critical texts is to overlook, or overwrite, the discursive complicity of how the authors view themselves semantically, how authors enact their authority through their writing, positioning themselves within narratives that themselves constitute material and extramaterial formations. This has its primary origin in the perceived subject–object split that drives Cartesian thought and its much-touted objectivity. The pieces of memoir I insert here are part of my methodological approach, one that intends to bring into view the fallibility and risk of this author's (my) engagement with subjects who do not command the benefits of normative human rights. I combine fictional and historical narratives within the ambit of a critical, effluent eye that is also occasionally avowedly autobiographical, so that my complicities may become apparent to the reader.

This is risky business, especially where inserting oneself into the story can be viewed as taking place and space and voice from the communities, marginal to normative human-rights life, in which I have lived and worked. But the desire of a reader or listener to read or hear an unmediated voice of the other through the work of a critic speaks to fantasies of knowing an original native, of getting through to an "authentic" otherness, as though one can write with an invisible hand. Postcolonial identifications of the exotic understand this desire properly as an essentialist, imperialist fantasy. Any unmediated access to the other is always such a fantasy.

At issue is the assumption of effacement of author, of the privileged self, as a virtue in multicultural, diverse interactions. This is in the first instance contradictory: why would the best approach to establishing intersubjectivity, the relations between different subjects, be denial of one of those subjects? In any event, denial of subjectivity is a ruse: the presumption that one can deny one's being and the implications of one's values is the other side of the coin faced by the liberal gesture of inclusion, in which one "grants"—that is, assumes one is in a position to "give"—the minority subject rights, a space to speak, a voice. What is truly challenging in interracial, inclusive, gendered, and other forms of intersectional interaction in the colonialist-capitalist world is not a faux intersubjective communication based on an impossible negation of self or the instantiation of the liberal self as the generous accorder of space, rights, voice. It is the fraught business of genuinely intersubjective communication across radical difference, which cannot take place without risk, error, and subsequent recalibration.

I learned this from women I worked with in Soweto in the 1990s. I wanted to work with abused women there who would have been considered working-class within the harsh constraints of apartheid economics, who would be now in their nineties by age cohort: teachers, nurses, educated women who were the unacknowledged powerhouses of their respective families. The women were quite obviously and understandably tired of researchers "coming from the university to get their stories." Using a mutual friend, the author Miriam Tlali, as an intermediary, they invited me to write a life narrative of my own, which they would use to decide whether they would enter into a working relationship with me. They did not want credentials, which in the first instance I gave them and they rejected; they wanted from me what I had asked of them. So I sat down to write about myself with as little credentialism and academic authority as I could muster, no doubt faltering here and there. As I have noted previously, they responded sympathetically to parts of my narrative that they viewed as testimony to a somewhat difficult life. I was astonished, because I never thought, as a racially privileged, antiapartheid, white South African, that I had the right to view my life that way. These women were treating me to the status of a subject, the status that had eluded them most of their lives. This is when I learned that intersubjective communication across radical difference is not a zero-sum game, a question of denial of one side or another, but an opportunity plagued at times by mistakes, messiness, and misunderstandings, followed by recalibration and assessment, all along the way. Another set of fellow travelers who taught me this were all the doctors I met during the HIV work who had lived as students at Alan Taylor when I was there as a child. Our reminiscences over its space, air, and architecture were marked by a kind of hysterical, comedic, and intimate sharing of its awfulness. (We all remembered cement blocks and curling linoleum floors, decades past their due date.)

Bear with me as I explore this radical reciprocity in the context of an effluent eye, one that seeks to trace nonnormative subjects across species boundaries with a view to human right-making, as opposed to human rights. I define these terms in the following introduction. For now, suffice it to say that I am ecstatic that the gift of growing up weirdly, encountering a range of subjects not considered as subjects within the makings of the international, anthropocentric human-rights regime, let alone the sovereign state, has enabled me to develop the effluent eye.

Among the companions it is my pleasure to acknowledge are my siblings, Ann Jolly and John D'Aeth, who keep me attuned to the realities of infectious-disease surveillance and global "peacekeeping," respectively, in the face of state governance structures, and remind me of the value of our shared, uncanny childhood. I thank my intrepid companion on weird journeys since 1978, Philip Grobler, from kicking lampposts in Bloemfontein in the seventies to attending concerts in Fez this year. To the ridgebacks, Thabo and Woza, and their cousin, the labrador Ebony (who tolerates Woza's entirely mystifying fear of water), thanks for being sanity-making. Researcher friends of the HIV years, Alan Jeeves and Nomusa Mngoma: you were there and remained with me throughout. I am grateful to Derek Attridge, David Attwell, John Coetzee, Dorothy Driver, and the much-mourned Margaret Daymond and Margaret Lenta, for your unwavering ethical commitments in fierce times, and your generosity with my younger, often graceless self.

Thanks to the African Feminist Initiative at Penn State, particularly the elegant, sharp, loving, and enduringly generous Gabeba Baderoon, who midwifed this book; to Dorn Hetzel, for all the dog walks and talks through good and bad times; to Imran Jardine, for saffron tulips, food, and comfort; to Charlotte Eubanks, for her persistence in all things "yummy," including trust and our friendship; to the Bodymapping colleagues Antjie Krog, Courtney Kiehl, Molly Appel, and Hyunji Kwon—what a journey! To Sarah Clark Miller, Jill Engle, and Mark Brennan, of the gender-based violence prevention research cluster, thanks for your affection and patience. To the magnificent Carey Eckhardt and the inestimable Patrick Deane, without whom I would not have come to Penn State, my utmost gratitude. To the delightful Department of Comparative Literature colleagues, graduate students, and faculty alike, much thanks. Thanks especially to Bob Edwards, whose support during the writing was endearingly unrelenting; to graduate-student colleagues Hanan Al Alawi, Tembi Charles, and Amy Omolo—you teach me all the time. To Alex Fyfe and Ivana Ancic: you are phenomenal researchers, supporters, friends. To Victoria Lupascu, for your advocacy in times of others' illness, bravo! To Julie Salverson, writer and theater-for-engagement expert extraordinaire ("the half has not been told"), and Yazir Henri, whose ethics of violence and testimony keep me grounded in the post–Truth and Reconciliation Commission decades, you are both amazing.

To our Lake of Bays summer-loving family, Joe, Kelly, Ryan, Courtenay, Dillon, and Otis, to friends Sean and Arlene Dwyer, and to Trish for cottage hospitality, I can only say that childhood friendships of one's partner are priceless. To my Australian hosts, Rosanne Kennedy and Gillian Whitlock—insights the 2009 Canberra trip gave me made their way here; and to Jeremy Martens, the Institute for Advanced Studies and the Forrest Hall at Perth, all at the University of Western Australia—I finished the book while with you. To our Covid-19 family, the Karako-Besettes, how could we have coped without family dinners? To Rick and Robin, our global South kin—thank you. And to our Cape Town family—Gill Jordan, best of caregivers to the infant Rose and substantive editor most expert (what a combination!), Gerry, Pippa, Nan on the other side and Heidi—the summer days at Spinnakers are perfect: I would *never* have paraglided off Lion's Head without your prompting! For all the horses that have borne me and with me over the decades, from Nyane and Mohale in Mantsonyane to the beautiful beings twirling at Next Level Horsemanship in Center County, Pennsylvania, I am so grateful. To Chris Whynot and Josh Figlin, for working on my "hard-wiring" for decades: I couldn't have, would not have, persevered without you both.

I acknowledge the financial support of the Weiss family. It has been my privilege to have held the Weiss Chair in Literature and Human Rights and its generous resources for a decade. To Doug Armato, who believed in this book when some thought I was mad/bad; to Rosemary Hennessy, who was instrumental in making it work; and to anonymous reviewers and MBK, the most meticulous of copy editors, my thanks. Finally, to Henry Bolognaise: In the effluent world, you are soaring, riding the winds over the Drakensberg, where boundaries are simply irrelevant.

Introduction

Human Rights don't work for most humans in the era of colonial capitalism. In his 2018 *Colonial Capitalism and the Dilemmas of Liberalism*, Onur Ince reflects on the "curious and curiously persistent" notion of the British Empire as a liberal empire of commerce, despite the violent acts of dispossession, slavery, and degradation that characterized its economy, most notably in the colonies (2).[1] I use the term "colonial capitalism" in the light of work on capitalism and territorialism, such as that by Ince and Giovanni Arrighi (1994), to foreground the fact that, as David Harvey puts it, "whether of an American, British or Chinese shape, all imperial undergarments of a capitalist expansion have a similar cut, namely, accumulation by dispossession" (cited in Povinelli 2011, 18). By insisting on colonial capitalism in the current era, I highlight the continuation of this conundrum, in which liberal democracy as a global ideal is constantly threatened by the structural and material violence required to feed global capitalism's aspirations to be, or at the least to be perceived as, of universal human benefit.[2]

What's more, normative human rights work hand in glove with global capitalist regimes. Normative human rights are ubiquitous in Western critiques. The human they describe has the power to disarm some of the moves made by certain forms of posthumanism to protect the environment and by postcolonialism to address the destructive legacies of colonialism that emerge in our contemporary world through colonialist-capitalist practices. Colonial capitalism refuses to acknowledge the impossibility of its genesis without colonial expropriation of land, slavery, and the continuance of the logic of slavery in the transformation of human rights into consumer rights and the possibility of being bought and sold.

The Problem of Human Rights in the Face of Decolonization

Many of us know that human rights don't work for the majority in the era of global capitalism, but we're at a loss to think through alternatives. It seems as if to give up on the ideal of human rights is to invite further erosion of human rights. However, few in need of normative human rights, outlined in the United Nations 1948 *Declaration on Human Rights* (UNDHR) and its amendments, can access them. To know they don't work for the majority who would benefit from their safeguards, and yet to rely on them to do so—that is, to tick off as done those who cannot command those rights because the rights exist on paper—seems at least hypocritical, and at worst structurally violent.

Hannah Arendt famously identified the crippling paradox that accompanies the concept of human rights as both the manifestation of the (supposed) ubiquity and universality of human rights but at the same time their guarantor. Writing about the condition of statelessness between World War I and World War II, a condition that is increasingly not a state of exception in the contemporary moment, Arendt points out that, if a human being loses his political status, he should, according to the inborn and inalienable "rights of man," come under exactly the situation for which the declarations of such general rights provided, whereas actually the opposite is the case. "It seems that a man who is nothing but a man has lost the very qualities which make it possible for other people to treat him as a fellow man" (1976, 300).

So those who should bear rights should not be in the position of pleading for such rights. When those who do not have rights seek recognition for rights, the fact is they must instantiate themselves as victims before the law to claim, paradoxically, the exalted position of the human, which was never supposed to have left them in the first place. As Arendt puts it here once again, "a man who is nothing but a man has lost the very qualities which make it possible for other people to treat him as a fellow man."

Such qualities, however, are not only not universally held, but also not universally believed to be what makes the human, as Sylvia Wynter reminds us (2003). They are based on a Western notion of the human that has a specific cultural development in the post-Enlightenment building of man as a subject-citizen who commands rights. They manifest an inherent bias that positions everyone and everything that is not embodied in that notion of "man" as outside the ambit of respect. Quality, in the context of the human, of human rights, then, refers not simply to characteristics, but also to a sense of superior quality. Further, this human does not represent the human; he is considered to *be* the human; and he is considered to be universally desirable. The values that inhere in human rights are historically, contextually, a part of a colonial narrative that shows up in contemporary life through capitalism's adherence to those values.

It is said of Western European and American colonialism that whites colonized with the gun in one hand and the Bible in the other, justifying the former with the latter. This has an analogy in contemporary human-rights regimes, in which human rights are often used to justify supposed humanitarian interventions that are in fact undertaken with a view to acquisition of property through dispossession, either for the state itself or on behalf of its allies. (An example of this, the Australian Northern Territory Emergency intervention, is examined in some detail in chapter 5.) Following Wynter's calling out of what she has termed the "genre of man," this book argues for the unsettling of the "genre of the human" in which "human rights" are invested, and the calling out of the containment of the human by the *genre* of the human, which is aligned with but extends further than Wynter's "genre of the human as man," which I shall unpack shortly. Let me address the elephant in the room first: Why would anyone want to attack human rights?

The unsettling, or estrangement, of human rights may feel risky, because human rights comprise one of the most globally recognized conventions for an ethical sense of what it means to be human, even if that sense does not translate into adherence to the UNDHR and its amendments in actuality, and even though the concept of the human expressed in the declaration is consonant with colonialism. However, *there is risk in not unsettling normative human rights, too.* If there is no estrangement of normative human rights, there can be no thinking about what exceeds the human in its normative sense, no concept of that which I term the "effluent."

"Man," then, is not all humans. "Man," following Wynter, rejects or conveniently overlooks the practices of slavery and the accumulation through dispossession of Indigenous land that got capitalism going in all its settler lineaments, and the exploitative labor practices that sustain it today. This "Man" undertakes to represent, or in Wynter's terms, to "overrepresent," those outside of Himself to Himself, meaning that, to Him, there really is no outside-of-Himself. Planetary wellness, it would seem, will not prevail without colonialist-capitalist "Man" acting on the call to disintegrate "His" toxic self-regard. The fact that Man is included in the threat of extinction is of no comfort, for without interruption, He determines not only His own extinction, but also that of the co-constituted subject: the human, the nonhuman animal, and the "environment" in relation.[3] Effluence, as an extra-anthropocentric conceit, can drive the Anthropocene's denouement into narrative reach. The effluent eye interrupts Man's trajectory, making it a radically decolonial field of vision.

Why Do We Need the Concept of an Effluent Eye? What Is "It"?

Over the past three decades or so, criticism in various humanities disciplines has developed a literature of what Judith Butler calls the (un)"grievable," the precarious, that which is seen as valued-less or valueless, less worthy of care, or even a (human) burden (2006, 2009). Simultaneously, Black studies have generated metonyms of the cusp between land and sea, with specific investments in the transatlantic slave-trade history embodying Blackness. Butler's work may be seen to follow on the preoccupation in the 1980s with trauma theory that grew out of work on the Shoah/Holocaust. However, the movement toward the cusp, the border, and the littoral has at least some of its roots in Gloria Anzaldúa's 1987 work on the mestiza and "Borderlands" (of the U.S.–Mexico border) and, subsequently, in Wynter's identification of the concept "Western Man" (2003). "Western Man" incorrectly assumes himself to be the human carte blanche, with coloniality and whiteness embedded. What this hopelessly violent move obscures is its erasure of Indigenous, Black, mestiza, and biracial/multiracial consciousnesses, and with them, anticolonial care/love.[4] Recent explorations in Black studies articulate this denial, specifically invoking the littoral. What lies beneath the Atlantic—dead slaves and their affect, actuality, and surviving vivacity under normative conditions of Black death—are invoked in Christina Sharpe's 2016 *In the Wake: On Blackness and Being*. Tiffany Lethabo King's 2019 monograph on the frictions and contiguities of Native and Black epistemologies uses the shoal, as neither land nor sea, to figure the relations between obliteration through slavery, on the one hand, and Indigenous genocide, on the other. The effluent, I propose, has the potential to look through a specific lens to see the connection between Butler-influenced thought and the Black littoral. *The Effluent Eye* undoes Western Man, Wynter's "coloniality of being," through an attack on one of its most cherished mechanisms for "accommodating" the embodied persistence of Blackness, Indigeneity, and supposedly worthless being into the colonialist-capitalist order: "human rights."

I use what I call the effluent eye to reposition human rightness, to associate it with the rejection of the genre of "the human" that is central to normative Western "human rights," to propose a human right-making with the possibility for rights other than those. According to the *Oxford English Dictionary* (*OED* online), *effluence* means "a substance that flows out of something" or "the action of flowing out." I use the term to refer to that which exceeds the containment attached to the genre of the human: containment of the body by the brain, the state of its subjects and the power of human subjects over objects, as such containment is idealized in normative rhetoric of "human rights." It would be spurious to use the term *effluent* as if it did not carry connotations of sewage, waste, and toxicity beyond a generalized leakiness. *Effluvium* is related to effluence, in that *ex-*, *e-* and *ef-* all come from the Latin *ex*, meaning "out of," or "from." *Effluvium* is defined as "an invisible emanation," especially "an offensive exhalation or smell" or a "by-product, especially in the form of waste" (*OED* online). Effluent subjects are not in and of themselves waste or toxic in a fundamentalist sense. They may, however, be toxic to the normative sense of the human, and therefore to human-rights regimes.

My contention is that the site of potential toxic relationality between normative human rights and effluent being, brought into view by the effluent eye, is itself of worth, because it manifests human right-making. Right-making is not simply against normative human rights, it is beyond or outside of normative human rights. I focus on communities that cannot and do not command the benefits of human rights, and may not even want to do so. Deploying an effluent point of view, it becomes possible to see what the resources or capacities of such communities may be; the effluent eye makes methodologies for affirming alternative practices of human right-making possible.

I own, and own up to, the effluent eye here, and all the risks it entails, through the deployment of a specific methodology that constitutes the novel territory of extra-anthropocentric human rights, practices of right-making that reject the centering of the human as the unit of value that trumps all other subjects in the making of ethical being. Human rightness, I propose, is achieved in practice in the absence of human dominion as the ideal. The art of governing oneself and others in forms of imperial containment, be it containment of the body by the intellect, containment of objects as instruments of human "development," or containment of nation through sovereign-state decisions of inclusion and exclusion as humans are wont to do, is not an art of right-making, but an art of imperial forms of governance. This assertion is not a denial of the human, but quite the contrary. It is a setting of humans in relation to other forms of subjectivity, such as nonhuman animals and the environment, where the latter comprise a set of subjects in and of themselves. We cannot know these subjects intimately through an anthropocentric lens, but neither can we deny the relations we have with them because they are not human-like. Tracing these extrahuman relations is a step toward demythologizing human dominion in the making of human rightness.

What, then, do the effluent eye and effluent being look like? What is our subject? I embark here on an exercise in description that will be, I hope, a useful outline whose dimensions will be robustly demonstrated in the chapters that follow this introduction. The outline may look at times like a characterization or a phenomenology, but it is neither. A characterization presupposes an identification, and a "phenomenology" presupposes the possibility of "science . . . concerned with the description and classification of its phenomena, rather than causal or theoretical explanation" (*OED* online).

The effluent is not a subject in the Saussurean sense; "it" does not conform to the subject of semiotics, or of Louis Althusser or Michel Foucault. "It" is not even appropriately referred to by that pronoun, although that is the best I have here to stand in for the effluent. The effluent has subjectivity but not identity. "It" is emergent and decomposing, or decaying, and is never fully graspable as an identity fixed across time. The effluent comprises processes in which the emergent can be the decaying and the decaying can be the emergent. The effluent is a prophetic and poetic that is not able to be envisioned or controlled by the technologies of surveillance, of law, of subjectification.

Allow me a thought experiment in which I put W. B. Yeats's "Crazy Jane Talks with the Bishop" together with Marlene Nourbese Philip's 2008 *Zong!* Yeats's poem points to the effluent. Yet, because it affirms Crazy Jane's ability to respond, and indeed her response to the Bishop, it is contained within the realm of what Butler calls the "speakable": it is comprehensible as a lyric. Yet it is haunted by unspeakability, as Butler claims the speakable is:

> To move outside the domain of speakability is to risk one's status as a subject. To embody the norms of speakability in one's speech is to consummate one's status as a subject of speech. Impossible speech would be precisely the ramblings of the asocial, the rantings of the

"psychotic" that the rules that govern the domain of speakability produce, and by which they are continually haunted. (1997, 133)

In the Yeats poem, both the persona Crazy Jane and the entire lyric point toward the unspeakable but are contained within the speakable.

I met the Bishop on the road
And much said he and I.
"Those breasts are flat and fallen now
Those veins must soon be dry;
Live in a heavenly mansion,
Not in some foul sty."

"Fair and foul are near of kin,
And fair needs foul," I cried.
"My friends are gone, but that's a truth
Nor grave nor bed denied,
Learned in bodily lowliness
And in the heart's pride.

"A woman can be proud and stiff
When on love intent;
But Love has pitched his mansion in
The place of excrement;
For nothing can be sole or whole
That has not been rent.'" (Yeats 1989, 221).

Here we note that the poet grasps the fact that the effluent is not in and of itself toxic, or waste. Note the proximity between "love" and "the place of excrement" and between the "whole" and "the rent," the latter juxtaposing wholeness to the female body as commodity, or rentable, in the pun on "rent" as both that which is let and that which is torn asunder. Further, the Bishop's reference to the "sty" renders Crazy Jane a pig, in a proximity she affirms rather than denies. Yet the politics and poetics of the effluent are not valent in the poem, for Crazy Jane has a coherent voice: if the Bishop does not listen to her, that doesn't mean the reader/listener can't "hear" her. The Bishop and Crazy Jane are identifiable, discrete subjects involved in discourse. Readers are not in doubt about this as they read the discourse.

Philip's *Zong!* is a poetic sequence based on the *Zong* massacre. The captain of the vessel *Zong*, having apparently gone off course with slaves on board bound for the Dutch colony of Surinam in South America, determined that there was too little water on board for crew and slaves, and ordered the killing of between 132 and 150 slaves on and in the days following November 29, 1781. The historical record is famous and became even more so after Philip's publication and performance of her poetic sequence on the event. The owners of the *Zong* had insurance on the slaves and attempted to claim it, whereupon the insurance company refused to pay up, not on the grounds that the slaves were murdered, but on the grounds that the ship's company was not in danger of death by dehydration. The court records state that one slave managed to climb back on board, and some threw themselves overboard when they heard the cries of the others drowning.

Philip has three sources for her text: an ancestor's story, coauthored by Setaey Adamu Boateng; the extant record of the court case between the owners of the ship, the Gregsons, and the insurers, Gilberts; and the unnamed voice of one of the perpetrators. At first Gilberts were ordered to pay the indemnity for the slaves, but the subsequent case ascertained that the ship owners were at fault for hiring a captain who did not navigate correctly, and thus ordered the drowning of the slaves without due cause. The case records that the judges accepted the condition of slavery: "It has been decided, *whether wisely or unwisely is not now the question,* that a portion of our fellow creatures may become the subject of property. This therefore was a throwing over of goods, and of part to save the residue" (211; citation from the original case heard in 1783; emphasis added). The judges did not accept the claim of the necessity of the "throwing over of goods" due to the demonstrably poor condition of the ship and the evident and catastrophic failures of leadership in navigation and other decision-making processes.

Zong! uses the words of the court case as a word hoard to, as Philip puts it, tell the story that cannot be told. She takes the words from the court document to refer to the event in formations of the fugue, both in its musical form and in the form of the subject who has suffered a trauma and is amnesiac, not being able to recover themselves. The *fugue* is defined by the *OED* as:

1. Music

a contrapuntal composition in which a short melody or phrase (the subject) is introduced by one part and successively taken up by others and developed by interweaving the parts.
2. Psychiatry
a state or period of loss of awareness of one's identity, often coupled with flight from one's usual environment, associated with certain forms of hysteria and epilepsy.

Zong! is a "non-lyric." There is no consistent *I* or *you* through the sequence. The poems are incantations, with masses of space between the words, set as crests and bases of waves visually on the page, and bearing the (non)syntax of the underwater sound:

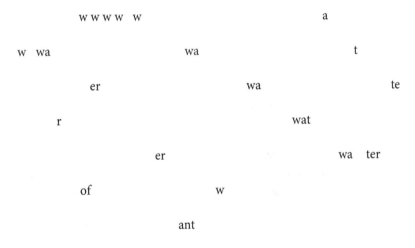

(from *Zong!* #1; 4)

As Philip-as-poet observes, and as at least one reader has observed, the (de)composed slaves decompose the subject, be it the *I*-who-writes or the *I*-who-reads. If the subject is in a fugue state, the body of the dead slaves cannot be exhumed, disinterred: the subject charged with doing that disinterring is itself reflexively rendered decomposed, incoherent. The poet writes in "Notanda" (the afterword in *Zong!*) that:

> The poems resist my attempts at meaning or coherence and, at times, I too approach the irrationality and confusion, if not madness (madness is outside of the box of order), of a system that could enable, encourage even, a man to drown 150 people as a way to maximize profits—the material and the nonmaterial. Or is it the immaterial? Within the boundaries established by the words and their meanings there are silences; within each silence is the poem, which is revealed only when the text is fragmented and mutilated, mirroring the fragmentation and mutilation that slavery perpetrated on Africans, their customs and ways of life. (195)

And this is the experience of (at least) one reader of the *Zong!* sequence:

> I think: it takes courage to keep reading; the courage to step overboard into meaninglessness has been stripped away; terror is deep. Philip is asking us to step overboard (willingly, we can choose) and experience the loss of what contains us (language, its rules, its customs), the safety of structures we've inherited—no, not safety, how dangerous it is to imagine that language is safe. I think: how language is set up in my guts and bones, how I have been taught (since I learned to read on Dick-and-Jane primers) to trust it, and how it lives in my skin (which is olive, but white for all intents and purposes) in my cells and nervous system, invisible, framing my points of view. Philip's own distrust of language forces her to pull it apart, to expose it, draw attention to its insides, to the stories/silences/murders/massacres that have been hidden there. (Klonaris 2011)

"Crazy Jane Talks with the Bishop" demonstrates Butler's speakable haunted by the unspeakable, where there is the grammar of the Dick-and-Jane primer, what Philip calls "the box of order" (2008, 192) that points to, but cannot admit of, its own incoherence. In the case of *Zong!*, however, the unspeakable is haunted by the speakable. The speakable cannot admit that the human cannot be slave. The impropriety of the fact that the human *is* a slave can be glossed within the speakable only as coincidental, relegated to a subordinate clause: "It has been decided, whether wisely or unwisely is not now the question, that a portion of our fellow creatures may become the subject of property." How to speak the unspeakable of the reality of the nonbeing of the slave as human becomes Philip's calling, her prophetic and poetic voice, in which the decomposed and the emergent coexist. Philip is a poet of the effluent, in large part because she consistently balances the ethical imperative to tell the story against the ethical imperative not to resurrect its enslaved victims as whole, to substitute for their violated being in an unscrupulous politics of body-snatching. Here "body-snatching" is my term for the practice of overwriting the dead, the violated, by presenting a fantasy of their health and well-being—their speakability as normative subjects—in the place of the ethical imperative to mourn-with (not to assume to be like) offered by the apprehension of suffering and dead embodiment. In an effluent reading, denials of the devastation wrought differentially on different places on land and in the sea and in space, and on distinct human beings and nonhuman animal beings, indeed form a practice of body-snatching. Such denials constitute a fantastic delusion of communal well-being.

Now I can return to a description of the effluent without, I hope, sounding too obscure, since the effluent is analogous to that which escapes our "regular box of order" or Butler's "unspeakable." Effluence has subjectivity, but is not a discrete subject and cannot therefore be fetishized. It can be, as we have seen, both emergent and decomposing, as in the effluent subjectivities of the *Zong*'s drowned, who emerge in the counter(f)actuality of Philip's poetics. It is a constellation of relations between humans, nonhuman animals, and the "environment," both alive and dead, where the environment is in scare quotes because it tends to be read as an anthropocentric word: that which surrounds humans, who are at the assumed center of it, is the environment. Effluent relations obtain in the energy of co-constitution through mutual care, or love. In a profound irony, the word *zong* is a mutilation of the Dutch *zorg*, meaning "care," the original name of the slave boat of Philip's poem (Webster 2007, 287).

Yet it is not a complete irony, for we cannot know what bounds of care persist in and on the *Zong*, from those who preferred to throw themselves overboard rather than see their companions drown alone, to Philip's loving fugue creation, *Zong!* The effluent is not an identity or character in and of itself. It is the relation between the sea, the drowned, and Philip (and even Philip's care to represent a perpetrator in the sequence) that brings the effluent constellation into emergence despite, or maybe even because of, physical decay. The effluent can be, and is, harmed by the sovereign state and colonialist-capitalist relations, yet it cannot be contained by the structural violence of those constructs. Even the writing out in the legal documents of human being as slave cannot control or censor the effluent subjectivity that emerges from Philip's poetics, in which humans' trajectory as slaves is not denied, but affirmed by entirely exceeding their status as such. Effluent being does not rely on the state and its associated apparati for care (say, the courts) and is often either entirely hostile to state sovereignty or regards the state anywhere on a scale from nuisance to irrelevant. The nation is anything but sacrosanct.

The effluent is not congruent with Butlerian disposability or the ungrievable because it has its own sovereignty and value, which is not that of colonial capitalism or the sovereign state. Indeed, I have argued, Philip's *Zong!* manifests a methodology and an aesthetics for grieving the ungrievable. The effluent is not productive of goods in the capitalist sense: it refuses the instantiation of the human as sovereign subject and object and refuses its attendant economics of commodification. This is one of the effluent meanings of those who were drowned and those who willfully followed them into the sea. The dead, in this context, end their commodification-as-slaves in the very act of dying.

The effluent may exceed the human and includes the human. However, it is not an all-inclusive company. The effluent is not naïve. It lives alongside colonial-settler imaginary, but is at home with itself. It is not an exotic looking for colonialist-capitalist converts or knowledge translation of itself into the ruins of, or ruinous, colonial capitalism. One can imagine, for example, how a superficial reading of the effluent could result in a seek and find of discrete "unspeakable" subjects that would then be fetishized for their supposed unspeakability, like so many Sarah Baartmans put on display for the normative, orientalist eye in a pornographic frenzy of liberal pity. Such pity is also a form of body-snatching, since the pity is seen to rehabilitate the subject of the spectacle, while instantiating the spectators as the generous accorders of the subjectivity at stake.

The effluent constellates its subjectivity through affirmation, not the politics of recognition. Liberal societies use recognition, as critics from Kelly Oliver to Alexander Weheliye have demonstrated, to accommodate those who claim to have suffered violence through expecting them to instantiate themselves (once again) as victims by begging those "valuable"/grievable within the hierarchy to recognize their suffering. Where "gross human rights violations" (GHRVs)[5] have been committed, survivors are often looking for recognition of the unimaginable, which belongs, categorically, to the realm of the unspeakable. Oliver (2001, 15) also uses Dori

Laub's formulation: to bear witness to ourselves, to develop an "inner witness," we need to have had experiences of ourselves as having been listened to, affirmed; we can see ourselves as valuable only if we have seen others seeing us as valuable. Elsewhere I have traced the mechanics of how witnessing before an authority that cannot see a victim as of worth can become an exercise in denial of worth. One sees the authority bearing witness to oneself—the victim-on-show—in a manner completely not coincident with one's sense of self. This creates traumatic fracturing in the very act that is supposed to "rescue." Can one explain effluent values to an authority, be it state or court, that cannot conceive of effluent value in the first place? What does it mean if the state has indeed inflicted GHRVs and it is to the state that one appeals for one's rights? Or, as a sexual assault survivor once put it to me in Soweto in 1996 (and I have heard several versions of this since working in the field of sexual assault care delivery), "how do you report police to police?" Ultimately, effluent subjectivity rejects the demands of normative human-rights regimes to instantiate oneself as a victim (again) to obtain rights one should have "enjoyed" in the first place but clearly did not; otherwise the violation would not have been, in the most practical of senses, doable.

The value the effluent creates and attracts is outside of colonial capitalism, involving Indigenous labor and embodied capacity outside the value of the normative subject as producer and/or consumer. In this sense, the confines of colonial capitalism produce threats to the effluent, not capitalism's proposed "necessity," which the effluent (literally and otherwise) does not buy. For example, categorically unrepaid subventions from Aboriginal lands and slavery were indeed "necessary" to get global capitalism going, but this does not amount to the necessity of capitalism, just as the fact that the court in the *Zong* case glosses over the decision to capitalize humans as immaterial does not render the question *settled*, to use the term in both its colonial and monetized terms.

I turn now to the question of *zorg* or care in the sense of health, in relation to the effluent. How the effluent constitutes care in relation to normative public-health assumptions is a preoccupation of this monograph. If the effluent eye can see bounds of care that are extra-anthropocentric, such a vision is not coincidental with normative public health, which assumes the physical well-being of humans and their survival as paramount. The difficulty this presents to the effluent eye is that such an eye can envision situations in which death is preferable to colonized or enslaved life. Some of us might not find surprising the acts of the slaves who jumped in voluntarily after their drowning companions in the *Zong* history, possibly owing to the unimaginability and distance of the event, in the sense that Oliver cites the "unimaginable" (2001, 1). Yet the unimaginability of the Indigene who is forced to "choose" between physical health and cultural death is constituted by the notion that settler colonialism is a healthy environment; and this is itself premised on the assumption that survivability in settler colonialism is always of benefit. So, for example, when I asked some doctors (not all!) in the Centocow region of KwaZulu-Natal (KZN) why they did not, or refused to, understand why HIV patients refused to take their highly active antiretroviral drugs (HAART) consistently, what lay at the heart of the matter was often the refusal of dual usage (of Western and traditional methods) as in any way beneficial, owing to the contamination of Western ideals with Indigenous practices, as well as to some youths' penchant for selling HAART in exchange for hallucinogenic alternatives. Bearing in mind that adult male unemployment for Blacks for the entirety of South Africa in the first quarter of 2022 was 38.6 percent, one has to ask: What, from the perspective of capitalist economics, do these young men coming from the remote, rural areas of KZN have in store for them? What, from a capitalist perspective, are they "saving themselves" for? This is a question I take up in detail in chapters 3 and 4. For the moment, however, it is sufficient to propose that the effluent eye affirms the emergent not-yet-subject, in this case youth who have not yet discovered their worth in non-capitalist terms, and whom the colonialist-capitalist view sees as always already waste before "it" (even) emerges as a vector of effluent subjectivity.

Public health, then, is not a good if the "public" in "public health" cannot affirm effluent being. Being effluent is not a state of cruel optimism. Effluent subjectivity living alongside colonialist-capitalist conditions has embodied knowledge that such conditions are harmful to effluent life. For example, effluent being might look like "spending time," as in wasting time in the sense of not producing capitalist value, but the very concept of spending time is nonsense within effluent being.[6] When effluent subjectivity, fragmented by colonial capitalism, is forced to view "itself" as spending time, as can happen (as when such subjects are assumed to be "lazy"), effluent subjectivity may well value physical self-harm as enjoyable, or even as a harm reduction strategy against colonial capitalism, as I argue in the final chapter. Effluent being embraces harm reduction rather than utopianism, optimism, or pessimism, because it lives alongside both possibility and extinction, to the point where they can be seen as one and the same within a range of ways to be. The effluent eye can see effluent subjectivity valuing being-with over surviving (like the *Zong* slaves who willed their own drowning) and valuing being per se rather than being like. For, "being like" is key to the triangulation that makes the possession of objects a competition between subjects to be wealthier than, to be more like, where "more like" indicates not a fixed goal, but a constantly desiring subject, which is capitalism's ideal and can be thought of as capitalism's object. Think, for example, of how the basic structure of desire in advertising is mimetic: we desire an object because someone else desires it as well. The fact that there is no object in the formulation "to be like" is the clue that being like has no fixed object in the endless desiring with no "enough," the endless desiring of objects that makes capital accumulation "work." This "work" is very different from the Indigenous and other forms of effluent labor that I explore in the following chapters. Before we get that far, however, let me outline why I see the human right to health as a doomed strategy for health in the current era.

The "Human" Right to Health: A (Failed) Containment Strategy

The United Nations High Commission on Human Rights (UNHCHR) dictates that the World Health Organization (WHO) constitution of 1946 envisages "the highest attainable standard of health as a fundamental right of every human being" (United Nations General Assembly 1948). The first problem is with the concept of health as an attribute of human beings exclusive of the environment. If you are already living in an area of environmental degradation, where fracking, for example, or bad air quality, undermines your health and you do not have the resources to move, any health care you may be able access is geared toward ameliorating the symptoms of degraded environment and is not a cure as such. Indeed, the UNHCHR and the WHO make their division between the "human" and a human-manipulated environment clear in their explanation that the words "the highest attainable" do not mean that humans have a right to be healthy, in part due to governments' inability to control directly "socioeconomic conditions."

Good health is influenced by several factors that are outside the direct control of states, such as an individual's biological makeup and socioeconomic conditions. Rather, the right to health refers to the right to the enjoyment of a variety of goods, facilities, services, and conditions necessary for its realization (Office of the United Nations High Commission on Human Rights, 2008).

Good health, the text implies, means people have an improved standard of life through capitalist labor and the goods it provides. There is no mention of the reverse: that being poor and having work could indeed degrade one's health through exploitative labor practices. Here, access to health as a right, as a concept, cannot comprehend intergenerational experiences of "environmental" contamination. Further, the exclusion of the state as playing a role in socioeconomic conditions, alongside genetic factors, naturalizes the state as "off the hook" where socioeconomic conditions are concerned, as though capitalism itself were as natural as genetic expression. (Of course, the UNHCHR shows its age in assuming that what it calls biological makeup cannot be manipulated.)

The implication is clear: settler-colonial capitalism is the implicit framework within which the human is thought of in the UNHCHR and its related documents. This means that the "inalienable" right to health is fundamentally linked to the right to work, where labor is registered as work within the capitalist system. Much labor is, therefore, not accorded the category of work. Indeed, Indigenous nonsettler populations, such as hunter-gatherers—think of Inuit in Canada or the Khoi-San in sub-Saharan Africa or Indigenous peoples in Australia—are often regarded as "lazy" (even though, when they do take up positions within capitalist systems, they have also been considered to be interlopers, in the wrong place, or "exceptional").

The absent concept in the U.N. approach is the environment, not as that which surrounds the Human and over which He has no control, but in terms of a co-constituted subjectivity that we can call the human, the nonhuman animal, and "inanimate" matter in relation. This absence is also evident in narratives addressing both the relation between human and nonhuman animal, on the one hand, and that between landscape and its abuse, on the other. Both elisions depend on the post-Enlightenment split of the human from that which is other to the human, or of subject from object. This split, a profound threat to the United Nations' stated goal of attaining equitable health services across race, class, and gender, depends on anthropocentrism, where anthropocentrism refers to a human-centered, or "anthropocentric," point of view. In philosophy, anthropocentrism can refer to the point of view that humans are the only, or primary, holders of moral standing. Anthropocentric value systems thus see nature in terms of its value to humans. While such a view might be seen most clearly in advocacy for the sustainable use of natural resources, even arguments that advocate for the preservation of nature on the grounds that pure nature enhances the human spirit must also be seen as anthropocentric (Padwe 2013).

Here we can begin to see that the anthropocentric view and the subject who inhabits the UNDHR coincide. However, radical critique in terms of both the character of the subject in the UNDHR and the subject of anthropocentrism demonstrates that the subject in each case refers not to all humans, but to what Wynter calls the "genre" of the human or the genre of "being human" (2003, 269). The problem of the Human of the Anthropocene is the same as the problem of the genre of man in Wynter's work, which has its roots in the Fanonian critique of European Man. To reprise the dilemma in Arendt's terms, those who should bear rights (Mankind) should not be in the position of pleading for such rights. When those who do not have rights seek recognition for rights, as I noted earlier, they have to instantiate themselves as victims before the law, paradoxically, in order to claim the exalted position of the Human, which was never supposed to have left them in the first place.

The values that inhere in "human rights" are historically, contextually, a core part of colonial narratives that emerge in contemporary life in capitalism's adherence to those values and in the fact that settler colonialism is not confined to history. Wynter emphasizes her own and others' exclusion from the category of the human on the basis of their race (Blackness) and their gender (not male): "Our struggle as Black women has to do with . . . the displacement of the genre of the human of 'man'" (288). Wynter proposes that, "because of this overrepresentation by the Genre of Man, which is defined in the first part of the title [of Wynter's article] as the Coloniality of Being/Power/Truth/Freedom, any attempt to unsettle the coloniality of power will call for the unsettling of this overrepresentation" (260). Wynter's use of "unsettling" means not just awkward or uncomfortable, but in my reading also refers to the colonial character of human rights. This colonial character of human rights has generated the imperial mode in which pandemics are thought of: the anthropocentrism, xenophobia, and lack of global rather than national scales of pandemic-talk are no match for twenty-first-century pandemics taking place in conditions of increasing "hypercapitalism."[7] Effluence, as a methodology that navigates between categories, rather than being addicted to them, is required instead.

Thinking pandemic through the lenses of the genre of the human and the national is radically inadequate. A further, related barrier to our concept of health obtains in the ways in which we live in the contemporary world. Fifth-wave public-health theory rejects framing health challenges that current, globalized communities face as events that can be addressed from within extant conceptions of public health. These challenges are best understood, fifth-wave public-health advocates argue, not as diagnoses, so much as symptoms of the unsustainable ways of living promoted by late-capitalist political, material, and sociocultural practices of being in the world. These ways of being and the (failed) promises attached to them form a "fifth wave" of public-health challenges, in which public-health interventions per se have diminishing returns in an environment in which the ways of being in the world to which late capitalism habituates humans are themselves the ailment, not the secondary "infections" they produce. Overwhelming poverty, substance (ab)use, malnutrition, overnutrition/obesity, and other stress-related illnesses have their drivers in working conditions and gaps between rich and poor. Or as Peter Hanlon and his coauthors put it, a "fifth wave" in public health is necessary to address these health issues, which are occurring in a context where society is also facing challenges created by "the broader problems of exponential growth in population, money creation, and energy usage" (2011, 30). In this context, as with environments directly damaged by extractive ecologies, accessing health is more likely to mean harm reduction than cure, since one cannot live outside of colonialist-capitalist damage, even if it is affecting one's health negatively.

This changes our reading of character from the well-worn narrative path of assessing individual moral failures and virtues to one of affirming persistence[8] in the face of the structural violence of global capitalism. Even more radically, in some instances, such persistence can mean availability to be harmed in situations where the choice not to persist may be seen as preferable to sustaining life. Indigenous communities such as that depicted in Alexis Wright's 2006 epic *Carpentaria* (Waany/gi communities of the southern part of the Carpentaria Peninsula, Australia) do not read substance abuse and self-harm as inherently pathological, a series of "bad choices" on the part of individuals.[9] I address questions of substance use in the settler colony in chapter 4 and explicate *Carpentaria* as an exemplary right-making artifact in chapter 5. For the moment, let me observe that the model of character that reads health as a personal responsibility and outcome, as is the case in the conventional bildungsroman and its mutually sustaining narrow medical model of morality, glosses over inequitable living conditions as an aspect of fate. This model ignores health-choice disablement[10] among Indigenous populations. *Carpentaria*, among other works of fiction dealing with Indigenous health in settler contexts, suggests that the cult of individual choice is a complicit practice, enabling ignorance of the construction and conditions of residential school experiences and labor for Indigenous peoples as both racist and a trajectory of harm.

Access to heath as a right cannot correct intergenerational experiences of "environmental" (including climate change) or settler-induced exploitation or slavery or their intersection, which sit at the nexus of vectors of harm. Extractive industries' exploitation of land and both nonhuman and human animals is part and parcel of the same coin. Further, since national and international organizations motivate for such exploitation, they too can be described as extractive industries. Black Lives Matter strikes a chord (or discord) precisely because, within Wynter's "genre of man," Black lives are perceived as matter: and those who have lived as Black/Brown matter and those of us who bear conscientious witness to that nonmattering know it and explicitly acknowledge it.

Effluent thinking that enables a decolonial context for viewing the relations between history, disease, human and nonhuman animals, and the "environment" equips us to understand the pandemic phenomenon in all its complexity. Here I give a (very) brief rehearsal of the geneses of HIV, SARS-CoV (Severe Acute Respiratory Syndrome Corona Virus), and 2019-nCoV, concentrating on the case of HIV because we have a good historical sense of its trajectory, to underscore this point. The question of a decolonial history of medicine is the central topic of chapter 2. Here I touch on that history to contextualize the need to reject the category of Man in reading pandemic disease and to instantiate what I call the effluent eye in its stead.

HIV has its genesis in the Kinshasa region, between 1910 and 1930, when the virus jumped the species boundary from its simian origins, initially probably because of bush hunting. (The reservoir populations of HIV are the red-capped mangabey [*Cercocebus torquatus*] and the greater spot-nosed monkey [*Cercopithecus nictitans*]; the transmission species is chimpanzees [*Pan troglodytes*], who prey on monkeys.) What drove its spread, however, was the rapid growth of Leopoldville, which was under the direct, personal ownership of Leopold II of Belgium up to 1908 and was subsequently a Belgian colony until 1960. Indentured laborers were being captured to produce rubber, railways were built, sexually transmitted infections were high (at one point, Leopoldville had a male to female population ratio of 2:1), and public health campaigns inoculating natives against diseases such as sleeping sickness involved the reuse of needles. (The inoculations had to do with keeping a labor force active, rather than concerns over the population health of native families as a social unit.) The setting was the perfect storm for a virus migrating from its reservoir population in the south of the Congo to Kinshasa and subsequently to Brazzaville up the river.

As Oliver Pybus and his fellow authors point out, "despite the importance of geography for infectious disease epidemiology, the effects of global mobility upon the genetic diversity and molecular evolution of pathogens are under-appreciated and only beginning to be understood" (2015, 1). In 2003, I was about to start work with colleagues in South Africa on the HIV/AIDS and gender-based violence (GBV) project. Our "kickoff" meeting was held in the Toronto area. Much to the surprise of some of us, the South African contingent's supervisor, Eleanor Preston-Whyte, was reluctant to let them attend, because Toronto was the locus of a spiraling pandemic at the time. (The surprise shows just how biased the global North and West is about perceiving disease as generated in the Global South, rather than "at home.")

SARS-CoV first appeared in China's Guangdong province in November 2002. On March 12, 2003, the WHO issued a global alert, warning of atypical pneumonia spreading among hospital staff. Three days later, WHO named SARS and put out an emergency travel advisory: the disease was spreading throughout the world by people using air transport. The areas affected included, at different moments, Hong Kong, Toronto, several areas of mainland China, and Taiwan. Horseshoe bats are suspected to be the reservoir species of SARS-CoV, although masked civets are identified as the transmission species to humans, possibly in wet markets.

Since 2003, there have been four small outbreaks of SARS. However, the WHO warns that "these events demonstrate that the resurgence of SARS leading to an outbreak remains a distinct possibility" (2003). In January 2020, a novel coronavirus, SARS-CoV-2, was identified as the cause of an outbreak of viral pneumonia in Wuhan, China. The disease, later named coronavirus disease 2019 (Covid-19), subsequently spread globally. In the first three months after Covid-19 emerged, nearly 1 million people were infected and 50,000 died. It is relatively clear that bats are (once again) the reservoir species for SARS-CoV-2, but we do not yet know what the transmission species to humans is: it could be bats themselves or, as is more likely, an intermediate species, or sets of intermediate species. Bats have long been known as an important reservoir for many zoonotic viruses, including rabies virus, Hendra virus, Nipha virus, Ebola virus, St. Louis encephalitis virus, and the beta coronaviruses that cause SARS and MERS (Middle East respiratory syndrome). The key to both zoonotic (transmission to human) and anthroponotic (transmission to nonhuman animals from humans) prevention is to determine how reservoir populations, transmission species, and the infected interact to prevent the spread of infection. For example, it was originally thought that pangolins, the most traded nonhuman animals globally, may have been the transmitters of Covid-19 to humans. However, the virus in the pangolins reveals that their disease was transmitted to them by humans, probably while hunting, selling, or butchering the pangolins. Thus conclude the scientists:

> Our study suggests that pangolins are natural hosts of Beta coronaviruses. Large surveillance of coronaviruses in pangolins could improve our understanding of the spectrum of coronaviruses in pangolins. In addition to conservation of wildlife, minimizing the exposures of humans to wildlife will be important to reduce the spillover risks of coronaviruses from wild animals to humans. (Liu et al. 2020)

A similar train of thought on required research comes from those working on the pathway of SARS between bats, civets, and humans:

> The genetic diversity of coronaviruses found in bats highlighted our poor understanding of viruses in wild animals. . . . There is an increased possibility of virus variants crossing the species barrier and causing outbreaks in humans as people come into closer contact with wild animals. . . . It is likely that in the emerging path of SARS-CoV, there are still other species missing between horseshoe bats and masked palm civets. One way of revealing possible links and suspects is to look at the ecological circles of both bats and masked palm civets. Alternatively, constant survey of wild animal species for SARS-CoV-like viruses should provide further information on animal reservoirs. (Shi and Hu 2008)

In my 2020 and 2022 studies on the pandemic, I used the term "zoonoses" in scare quotes because a decolonial, nonanthropocentric approach enables us to see these zoonoses as actually reverse zoonoses or zooanthroponoses (passing from human to nonhuman animals) at the systemic level: that is to say, it is the role of Man in global "development" that has brought these diseases to bear through the concentration of human and nonhuman contact in zones under ecological stress. A successful vaccine for Covid-19 is merely a solution to the novel coronavirus that causes it; more will follow, precisely because the ecological stress on human and nonhuman environments is growing as the physical contact zones between species are shrinking. Human–nonhuman-animal–environment ethics are required to conserve the compound subject. Until these three subjects are understood as co-constitutive along lines of intimacy that materialize as both care and enjoyment, colonial capitalism and its cult of Anthropocentric fetishism cannot but result in ever increasing waves of "zoonotic," or rather anthroponotic, disease. But this requires thinking of the human as an effluent subject, rather than the logocentric "Man" that Wynter targets. Let us begin with this effluent eye and let us turn it on that categorization that most troubles logocentric Man's coherence: (His) death, or His dependence on body-snatching His and others' embodiment.

1

Effluence, "Waste," and African Humanism

Extra-Anthropocentric Being and Human Right-Making

In this chapter, I establish precisely what I mean by "normative human rights." I then bring an effluent eye to bear on normative human rights when describing the situation of communities that do not have access to normative human rights and for whom the state has never been a securer of those rights. The notion that such communities can appeal through the courts, national or international, for access to human rights is fantastical: not the communities' fantasy, but a fantasy of those, who are themselves already secure and think that the majority of people who do not command human rights can access them through legal procedures. The rare occasions on which such appeals are successful feed the fantasy of ubiquious access to human rights.

I use the effluent perspective to dislodge normative human rights to make room for their alternative "human right-making." Human right-making applies to relationships between humans, but also those between humans and objects and the environment, rather than the human as a subject in and of itself that constitutes the "overrepresentation" of the human, to use Sylvia Wynter's term (2003). The human in and of itself is an impossible subject from the perspective of the effluent eye, as the human is not self-sustaining and is, as a singular, imperial subject, predatory on its supports. Further, human right-making is, in the first instance, a set of actions and practices; it does not inhere in simply being for the sake of the human in and of itself. Moreover, I address the question of how the genre of the "human" has so imbued English with its values that trying to write in English about that which exceeds the genre, attempting to bring an effluent eye to English, is itself a formidable task.

At the heart of the matter is the existential problem that death poses for the genre of the human, in a way that it does not for effluent communities. To demonstrate an alternative, or effluent, approach to death, I use Es'kia

Mphahlele's reading of African humanism, which offers a way to grieve material being that is extrinsic to the lenses of both secure individual citizen and the state, where the state is conceived of as having both the ability and the duty to offer citizens security. I apply this approach to see what alternative subjectivities to those of normative human rights become visible. The scene of this unmasking is the mortality produced by the South African HIV epidemic. State-mandated rollout of highly active antiretroviral therapy (HAART) began only in 2003, did not undergo a growth spurt until 2008, and is still a project with significant challenges. I then return to the land of theory to demonstrate how neither posthumanism nor postcolonialism can conceptualize Mphahlele's take on African humanism. Its story is unspeakable in their liberal humanist terms, or in the terms of the overrepresentation of the human as sovereign subject.

Normative Human Rights and the "Human" Subject

The post-Enlightenment focus on the human as the proper subject of narrative is the anthropocentric property of the Western discourse of modernity. (I say "post-Enlightenment," as there are strains of pre-Enlightenment narrative that are nonanthropocentric, despite their Western origins, such as the Icelandic sagas.) In the preface, I talked about tracing the subjects of various kinds of narratives, fictional and nonfictional, as crucial to outlining human rights and the role they play in the entrenchment of colonialist-capitalist anthropocentrism, as well as their less omnipresent, but vital, persistent alternatives. The Human subject is the building block of post-Enlightenment narratives, to the extent His ubiquity constitutes an interdisciplinary genre of the human that ranges across legal, fictional, and historical narratives.

Joseph Slaughter proposes that the human rights conventions of the United Nations 1948 *Declaration of Human Rights* (UNDHR) and its related legislative conventions share with the novel, and in particular the bildungsroman, a subject (2007, 4). In both cases this subject is proposed as commonsensical and available to all; but the constitution of the subject requires the work of "literary and cultural forms" to make sense of human rights norms (6). The genre of the human is not an epiphenomenon of the essential human, then, but is *fictional,* having a character that itself can change. The very construction of character, its resistance and malleability—its vibration, as it were, in the face of seismic changes in our sociocultural fabric—has to be explicit for us to understand Slaughter's argument. That is to say, the subject of narrative discourse, be it explicitly fictional or nonfictional, is always, in its radical sense, invented: it manifests how we locate ourselves as subjects in performative rhetorical acts that actually do play a role in shaping our material environment. For example, if we perceive ourselves as humans, and that means (post-Enlightenment) that we are the embodiment of rational energy in relation to other forms of being, we put ourselves in a position to organize our physical environment around our needs and desires, even if these needs and desires result in negative consequences for that environment. Where does this power come from?

When we speak about the binary pairs such as the human–nonhuman, subject–object, culture–nature, and mind–body, the human is accredited intelligence akin to or, in the absence of G-d, as a creator and as master of his body, nonhuman animals, and his environment. Frantz Fanon explicitly introduces race into this picture, pushing the bourgeois European family unit and its gendered dynamics, as outlined by Freud, into the context of racialized colonialism (1991a; 1991b). Whereas Freud assumes the proper subjects of psychology to be the Viennese family at the turn of the century, Fanon (who himself trained at the Sorbonne and had all the power of a colonial elite, but not that of whiteness) exposes race as an indelible line: people who embody Blackness are associated with the animal, rather than the human. With the explicit posing of race as the scene of the subject comes a nonhuman menagerie in its worn-out animality, assigned in excess to the racialized other, with the Black-as-monkey being a preeminent example.

This racialized figuration of that which is other to the bourgeois, human subject of dominant forms of the novel and the UNDHR demands a rethinking of what I call the waste(d), wasteful, or effluent subject in relation to the normative subject described in Joseph Slaughter's 2007 *Human Rights, Inc.* The human subject, as it is discursively located in the Western traditions of the novel, and in the attendant genre of the human in legal terms, is subtended by the otherness of the female, the Black, and the nonhuman other, be it considered animate (nonhuman animal) or inanimate ("natural" or manufactured "object") within the genre of the human. The challenge, then, as stated by Claire Jean Kim, is as follows:

> Rethinking the human begins with the recognition that the human has always been a thoroughly exclusionary concept in race and species terms—that it has only ever made sense as a way of marking who does *not* belong in the inner circle. It means clarifying that the project before us is not an *extensionist one* (expanding the definition of the human to allow a few radicalized groups or preferred ape species in) but rather a *reconstructive one* (reimagining humans, animals, and nature outside of systems of domination). (2015, 277; emphasis original)

Just as capitalism has demanded subventions from slavery and its related histories of exploitative labor practices, the idea of the "human" as character in the Western genre of the human has achieved its liberal humanist manumission, so to speak (tellingly self-accomplished!), by the enslavement of the female, Black, not-white/nonhuman, nonhuman animal, or disabled other. This complex is rendered as a conglomerate, a set of effluent objects in the view of the human subject Kim outlines. This human subject is also a colonialist capitalist. Think of the capitalism central to the fictional moment that Daniel Defoe's *Robinson Crusoe* marks with such explicit productivity. Defoe links colonialist-capitalist and related enterprises to modernity's designation of any activity that does not contribute to capital accumulation as waste, or wasteful. Crusoe is the exemplary colonialist capitalist. And Friday is wasted, unable to enter into full personhood until Crusoe harnesses his energy for production. Hunter-gatherers such as Friday are lazy, from the colonial perspective of the bildungsroman, and certainly not eligible to be protagonists.

Slaughter contends that the bildungsroman is a preeminent manifestation of human rights in postcolonial settings. Marianne Hirsch, among others, claims that "the *Bildungsroman* continues to serve . . . as 'the most salient genre for the literature of social outsiders, primarily women or minority groups'" (cited in Slaughter 2007, 27). I disagree. It continues to serve as the most apprehensible genre to those inured to reading within the genre of the human; it is not necessarily the most salient genre for "minorities," a term that does not satisfy my desire for specificity in the characterization of that vast variety of subjects rendered marginal to liberal human discourse in the first instance. Why is the most salient genre for such "minorities" inevitably the one in which "we" (a liberal, globalized/metropolitan reading public) understand "them" best? This brings us to the question of language. Those comfortable with the way in which the genre of the human has imbued contemporary English usage might well agree with Slaughter and Hirsch. But what if, as Marlene NourbeSe Philip proclaims, "English is a foreign Anguish?" (1989, 44–46).

You may have noticed that I am struggling to distinguish between the "human" of the genre of the human and simply saying human, which creates a kind of overblown but necessary wordiness in my explanations. This is a symptom of post-Enlightenment English's inability to deal with the distinctions between its values—"Man" and therefore human—and what those nouns might signify within a different cultural context. I use "genre of the human," following Wynter's use (2003, 269), to signal the possibility of such a change in context. Similarly, embodied spiritualities that fall outside the ambit of the binary of material–spiritual confound post-Enlightenment English, which can get at them only through words that suggest some sort of cult, like totemism and animism. Embodied spiritualities are extant, not in some pure precolonial and hence "primitive" form but as cultural practices that have been persistent in the onslaught of colonial capitalism and whose resilience is manifestly evident, as critics as various as Mark Rifkin (2012), Sam McKegney (2007), Elizabeth Povinelli (2011), and Wole Soyinka (1976) seek to explain, and as the non-Western cultures and writers they explore manifest.

The difficulty all these critics face (as I do) in using English to address cultures for whom the Cartesian subject–object split is not the central dilemma, except through a considerable colonial and neocolonial "inheritance," is that the words we have for such non-Cartesian ways of being are deeply embedded in their usage within Cartesian traditions. Hence, according to *Merriam Webster's Collegiate Dictionary*, in its 1995 edition, *animism* is defined as the belief that materials, such as natural phenomena, "have a consciousness" or as the "belief in the existence of spirits separable from [human] bodies." It is precisely because "English is a foreign Anguish," as Philip says, obsessed with maintaining the mind–body binary and its related values, such as the human–animal divide, that I cannot "just tell my story." I need to defamiliarize and unsettle the very terms that use the genre of the human at the same time.

Literary criticism and cultural studies more generally have critiqued the genre of the human in the forms of critical Black studies, radical feminisms, environmental criticism, and disability studies, while posthumanism and new materialism, in their intersections with the former approaches, attempt to address the subject in excess of the liberal humanist tradition. The question, then, is to what degree these attempts to deconstruct the genre of the human are still "stuck" in the modes of conceiving of the human and its excesses within the Western genre of the human.[1] Specifically, how does this addiction to the human continue to generate categories of second- or third- or fourth-class (non)citizens as waste: wasted humans, wasted materials, wasted beings that together constitute subjects of effluence within my framework? The narratives of *effluent* communities, of which my first example is Mphahlele's proposed but unwritten story, prospectively entitled *And the Birds Flew Away* (Samin 1997), never assumed the genre of the human to be their norm or their habitus. This is not due to "human rights" positioning effluent narratives as inferior (which is indeed the case), but to the irrelevance of *those* rights to effluent subjects in terms of actually accessing rights and to the inability of human-rights regimes to comprehend nonanthropocentric forms of the imagination required for human sustainability. Perverse, but true. To understand how to make the human sustainable, we need to figure out how to decenter the human. Zakiyyah Iman Jackson asks, "Might there be a posthumanism that does not privilege European Man and its idiom?"

Posthumanism's past (and arguably ongoing) investment in Europe as standard bearer of "Reason" and "Culture" circumscribes its critique of humanism and anthropocentrism, because it continues to equate humanism with Enlightenment rationality and its peculiar representation of humanity, "as if it were the human itself" (2013, 673).

What Jackson means by enlightenment rationality is precisely what I talked about earlier in terms of containment and dominion. But the Enlightenment is a historically specific Western phenomenon, not universal, as Jackson points out. So, even posthumanism, she contends, while it seeks to underscore the need for humans not to perceive themselves as the center of the universe, cannot accomplish its goal because it cannot relinquish the genre of the human. In other words, posthumanism is in trouble because it tries to deny its own complicity in the value of the "human" of "human rights" while simultaneously trying to decenter that human. Jackson concludes with another question: "Is it possible that the very subjects central to posthumanist inquiry—the binarisms of human/nature, animate/inanimate, organic/inorganic—find their locus outside of the epistemological locus of the West?" (2013, 673). My answer would be a resounding Yes.

The Inadequacy of Postcolonialism and Disposability to the Effluent

Before we get to what subjects look like outside the "epistemological locus of the West," I address the limitations of two key areas of criticism that claim to address, or even in cases redress, the binary categorizations that Jackson lists, but are for the most part too addicted to the genre of the human to do so: postcolonialism and Butlerian theories of disposability.

Pathological Postcolonialism

Neil Lazarus argues, in an interview with Sorcha Gunne, that the field of postcolonial studies is itself a product of the poststructuralist moment, which creates what he calls a "wrong turn" for the discipline (Gunne 2012, 9). That is to say, the focus on discursive play and the features that a certain kind of postcolonialism fetishizes as quintessentially characteristic of a predetermined *essence* of the postcolonial approach stem from a literary-critical academy too attuned to poststructural play to address the vast exclusions this orthodox "postcolonialism" entails.[2]

Lazarus says: "I've always wanted to read against ... a certain approach that favors decenteredness, catachresis, instability, ambivalence, the migratory, the diasporic, the in-between, etc. ... The 'pomo-postcolonialist' tendency has led to a hypostatization of certain formal aspects in literary works (self-consciousness, contingency, a stress on incommensurability and the failures of language to signify, etc.) whose one-sidedness again seems to me narrow and impoverishing" (Gunne 2012, 5).

The attention to deconstructive form in the postcolonial canon selected for its amenability to what Lazarus calls "pomo-postcolonialism" is what I call "pathological postcolonial criticism," because it seems to assume, falsely, that the *deconstructive artifices it fetishizes* equate to the *disassembling of the genre of the human* in ways consistent with the *disassembling of colonial and neocolonial structures* at the level of textual politics. Such pathological reading does not deconstruct the colonizing and colonized human, but simply caricatures the human per se as deluded unless humans, whether colonized or colonizing, "understand" they are at the mercy of poststructuralist play. The pathology lies in the delusion that the cynicism of poststructuralist play marks, rather than masks, material practices of colonization, capitalism, and related forms of tyranny. In this sense, poststructural play can be seen as a recognition of structural violence that masks its impact by divorcing the rules of the game from questions of political power, or at the very least suggests that most citizens are either unaware or incapable of countering such power, or both. It is, of course, only those who have the benefits of commanding human rights who can write off the project of human rightness as fundamentally, necessarily lodged in bourgeois character production and anthropocentrism.[3]

Lazarus identifies 1975 as the moment at which former radical connections between the West and third-world struggles for anticolonialist nationalisms and self-determination fell prey to the period of postwar austerity (and its attendant crises) that oversaw the installment of neoliberal regimes and entrenched neoconservative ideologies. Thus, when I read *The Meaning of Contemporary Realism* by Georg Lukács (1962) as a child in South Africa in the early 1970s (because my mother was teaching it at the then University of Natal, Durban), and when I diligently read Georg Gugelberger's *Marxism and African Literature* when it first came out in 1985, both texts seemed to me bizarrely ahead of themselves in terms of their political concerns and also strangely behind, or at least outmoded. To some degree, as Lazarus highlights, the focus on poststructuralism and postmodernism in the Anglo-American academy, rather than the more radical strains of anticapitalism and anticolonialism, does more than simply "write off" preexisting forms of anticolonialism prematurely, arguing as it does for the "collapse," the "exhaustion" and "the falsity of that earlier moment" (Gunne 2012, 10); it also detracts from a sustained history of colonialism across the twentieth century, including the U.S. forays into Iraq and Afghanistan (Gregory 2004).

Pathological postcolonialism insists on the failure, belatedness, and "falsity" of movements such as the international anticolonialist and antiracist alliances that resulted in Russian-backed Cubans fighting heavily against the illegal South African occupation of then South-West Africa and its equally illegal war in Angola to maintain a boundary of white power. This skepticism has left Anglo-American pathological postcolonialism with a skewed version of history, one that has jettisoned materialist readings in favor of the deconstructionist location of poststructuralist play. Its capacity for endless identifications and analyses of imperialist power offers little sense of the postcolonial subject as *that which exceeds its victimization by colonial power,* in terms both of that subject's knowledge of worlds in excess of Western epistemologies and of that subject's manifestations of persistence in the face of—rather than resistance to—colonial and neoliberal powers.[4]

Here, I critique specifically postcolonial resistance conceived of as that which opposes an assumed neocolonial and neoliberal norm within the Manichean imagination of a "writes back" postcolonialism. This is a temporally limited move that relegates that which is incidental or external to a set of privileged archcolonial moments, surplus to the "struggle at hand" and thus wasted effort. However, pathological postcolonialism is not a solution to the temporal conundrum of "writes back" postcolonialism, in that its love affair with poststructural form confuses deconstructive artifice with the rejection of bourgeois subjectivity; and pathological postcolonialism certainly has no truck with any notion of orthodox human rights or their reenvisioning, since its (to some) comforting skepticism does not simply disallow rightness as excess, but stigmatizes it as wasteful: who could be so naïve as to think of human rights, let alone rightness, as a meaningful category in the current global moment? I include this observation because, firstly, I don't see the textual or postmodern turn in postcolonialism as having been necessary to the evolution of postcolonialism generally and, secondly, because I wish to highlight the poverty of pathological postcolonialism in relation to actualizing (even) anthropocentric human rights, let alone the extra-anthropocentric human rightness for which I am arguing.

The acceptance of capitalism as the product of necessity, rather than political allegiances of power in the period following World Ward II prosperity, renders many citizens victims of their delusion of the inevitability of current neoliberal regimes of power. Our relative inability to discern the nexus of relations between colonialist, neocolonialist, and capitalist forces as having a material history that has led to the current juncture speaks to the naturalization of history under the rubric of necessity. This aporia also impedes recognition of interventions that exceed resistance, defined as temporally limited, to include persistence, as a form of nonquiescent endurance, or persistence in human right-making, as I outline below.[5]

The marketing of consumer choice as being an exercise in agency and freedom is enabled by the myth of American equality, which assumes we all start from the same positions of power; and it reduces choice materially to the confines of choosing *how* to live within the neoliberal state, not *whether* to live within it. This question does not enter the parameters of the body politic, as the failure of Bernie Sanders's 2016 campaign illustrated.

Communities of effluence live within sight of, or on the margins of, "the good life" (Berlant 2011, 2), and/or they have recognized that the good life is not their "good life" at all.[6] What kinds of narratives do these communities produce that exceed the normative materiality of hypercapitalism, and are restructuring the genres of "human rights" into practices of human rightness accordingly?

Resituating Butlerian "Precarity" and "Grievability" in Relation to the Effluent

Judith Butler claims "precarity designates that politically induced condition in which certain populations suffer from failing social and economic networks of support and become differentially exposed to injury, violence, and death" (2009, 25). That state has, however, taught us that "to be protected from violence by the nation state is to be exposed to the violence wielded by the nation-state," and that "precarity . . . characterizes that politically induced condition of maximized precariousness for populations exposed to arbitrary state violence who often have no option but to appeal to that state from which they require protection" (26). In other words, "to rely on the nation-state for protection from violence is precisely to exchange one potential violence for another. There may, indeed, be few other choices" (26).[7] Further, Butler underlines that the human-rights framework cannot render life *not* precarious, since the only form of life the human-rights regime recognizes is one that has a status of a person: one who has the actual potential to be, or is involved in, the *business* of creating the good life, the symptom and diagnosis of which can be only that material reality which we recognize as possession. She also argues (and I agree) that the conditions of life are deeply interdependent. But this interdependence in Butler is anthropocentric; it does not explicitly involve dependence on nonhuman subjects.

I have been arguing that capitalism renders the interdependency that is the precondition of sustaining life invisible in the sleight of hand in which the choice to thrive is reduced to making the "right" choices, especially the right choices about what kinds of products are most likely to get one further up the corporate ladder of the business of the good life. This situation is made all the more *less* free if one's security is both granted and threatened by the state, in a situation in which the state is in fact complicit in the transitioning of the rights of the citizen to those of the rights of the consumer.

In this light we need to go a step beyond Butler's comments on the state in *Frames of War: When Is Life Grievable?*:

> Without grievability, there is no life, or, rather, there is something living that is other than life. Instead, "there is a life that will never have been lived," sustained by no regard, no testimony, and ungrieved when lost. The apprehension of grievability precedes and makes possible the apprehension of precarious life. Grievability precedes and makes possible the apprehension of the living being as living, exposed to non-life from the start. (2009, 15)

The question of *who grieves* is crucial here, and in the absence of the subject, one assumes that what Butler decries is the lack of recognition of the state in cases of ungrievability. However, effluent communities that live with embodied knowledge of precarity nevertheless create (and have created) forms of grievability that do not depend on the recognition of the state. Communities of the effluent live outside or on the margins of the state in its assumption of "the good life" as everyone's business. Many postcolonial communities, Indigenous, and those otherwise rendered marginal are resilient precisely because they *no longer or never did* believe in the authority and/or capacity of the state to provide *basic security*, let alone any "good life." Thus, effluent communities, as I describe them, *already* live always with a sense of the grievability created in the wake of the capitalist state, because that state *constitutively* renders any life not involved in the business of life, as defined by Michel Foucault (2008) and Matthew Huber (2014) and others after them, to the effluent categories of never-having-been-born, precarious or already dead, and/or "objects," following the instrumentalist logic of the state. Alternatively, effluent communities can extend the realm of grievability to these and other beings where the state cannot. The inability of the state to support conditions of flourishing for the effluent brings about an issue for Butler's construction: *one cannot assume that, because the state does not provide conditions of flourishing, and therefore of grievability, grief from and for the effluent does not exist.* While grievability for the effluent subject may not exist outside of pity in non-effluent communities, it may well exist as a constitutive element of desire, pain, and resilience *within* the effluent, co-constitutive subject. To respond to Butler: there is something living, or rather happening, that is other than "life," as we shall see.

I begin by returning to Jackson's question: "Is it possible that the very subjects central to posthumanist inquiry—the binarisms of human/nature, animate/inanimate, organic/inorganic—find their locus outside of the epistemological locus of the West?" (2013, 673). For the moment, let us reframe her question this way: What does it look like to view death with an effluent eye, one that is in excess of the human as it is conceived of by the Western genre of the human? Once again, some might argue that a Western-trained humanist looking at these traditions may do so with a purely exoticizing eye; yet once again, I argue that recognizing the limitations of the Western genre of the human is possible for a Western-trained academic.

Having lived and worked in multiple Black sub-Saharan African communities as a child, an adolescent, and an adult, I do not count myself as outside of the animist traditions in which I was raised and with which I have been concerned in my domestic and working lives. I am, as it were, bicultural, having been immersed in non-Cartesian traditions but trained as a postcolonialist within the Western academy.

Some cultures, then, never assumed the centrality of the human; they always already saw human being as in relation to, not as having dominion over, objects and the environment. In these cultures, the Enlightenment's human rationality and the splits of mind–body, self–other, and human–nonhuman are not perceived as that on which the authority of our humanity depends. This means that the death of the human is an event for mourning the transition from human to nonhuman being in those cultures, but is not a termination of being per se. We all mourn the loss of a loved one, but that is different from the existential crisis specifically human death poses to an Enlightenment mind, in which the death of the human threatens the death of the subject altogether, as only genre-of-the-human-conforming subjects and their human associates are considered rights-and-value-bearing subjects in the first place. Put flippantly, post-Enlightenment values are so anthropocentric that, if a human is not there to see the world, the world disappears, as it is not a subject without humans' constitution of it as such.

Mphahlele's African humanism exhibits a linchpin of sorts that can move us into understanding the effluent subject, which exceeds the human subject.[8] His conceptualization of African humanism offers us a movement from the subject who acquires material, the proper subject of colonial capitalism, to the subject that acquires the status of the material, and thus, in terms of the *genre of the human,* is in fact *immaterial,* beyond citizenship, not able to avail "it"self of modes of acquisition or rights of belonging.

Mphahlele's African Humanism

Mphahlele's exemplary practice of African humanism bears an apparent likeness to the genre of the human, but simultaneously breaks decisively with it through attention to the unborn, the ancestors, and nonhuman animals. In these nonproper or effluent subjects, we can trace a subjectivity of the effluent, and indeed even an agency.[9] This "split" is not a result of a split consciousness on the part of Mphahlele as a primary custodian and philosopher of African humanism; instead, the split appears because the embeddedness of the genre of the human in English, in its post-Enlightenment practices of anthropocentrism, weakens its ability to express the effluent subject and at present is possibly completely incapable.

His African humanism contains within it two characteristic aspects, one consonant with post-Enlightenment Eurocentric humanism and one that pulls away from that tradition. The first is the idea of the centrality and survivability of the human; the second is African humanism's attempt to reference, in English, long-standing African animist traditions of vast variety through the phrasing of the human being living in harmony with "his" environment.[10] Here, however, the point is very much the specific challenge posed to post-Enlightenment thinking by the widespread sub-Saharan African belief in the simultaneity of the unborn, the living, and the ancestors as populations.[11]

The unborn are those who have yet to live; but because they have yet to live, they are not yet to be grieved, even if the neoliberal postcolonialist state's inherited genre of the human regards them as immaterial. Simultaneously, the ancestors are the advisers, those who point out when life is not being lived by the living in harmony socially or environmentally, and who have to be appeased for such harmonious living to indeed be accomplished. The unborn and the ancestors are not citizens, but they are subjects who are the focus of hopes, anxieties, and yes, grievability—and they themselves grieve—despite their Eurocentric categorization as immaterial to the genre of the human.[12] As practitioners of effluent grief, they form a model of persistence in the face of the reduction of meaning perpetrated by the genre of the human.

For Mphahlele, the nonproper, effluent subject that post-Enlightenment English resists is embodied in the afterbirth. Within Mphahlele's telling of the proper relations between the ancestors, the living, and the unborn, in a 1997 interview with Richard Samin, the placenta plays a crucial role. In the practice of burying the placenta after the birth of a child, the afterbirth is transformed from that which is dirt or waste into that which constitutes a metonymical connection between the unborn, the newly living, and the ancestors (Samin 1997). This is not "animist materialism" at work in Harry Garuba's (2003) sense of the term, in which objects are continually and renewably imbued with the spirituality of gods through metaphor. The placenta in Mphahlele's reading was never just an object, so no "continual re-enchantment of the world" (265) needs to take place. It is, in fact, precisely the placenta's nonfigurative, but material, metonymical[13] role in co-constituting relations between the unborn, the living, and the dead that garners "it" the extra-anthropological agency of the subject, where the subject is the effluent community whose proper noun would be something like "unborn-living-ancestors-earth."

Mphahlele, in part due to his deep understanding that a discursive move under apartheid to associate the white with the inhumane,[14] as both a political and aesthetic act, would merely rehearse post-Enlightenment's assignation of negative value to the Black in a reversal of poles, rejects Négritude (along with, most famously, Wole Soyinka) in favor of what seems like universal humanism under the title of African humanism: "There's a kind of piety also on my side that says to me no matter what human beings will survive and there is something intrinsic in the human species to survive" (Samin 1997, 185).[15]

However, when asked by Samin at the very same time about the meaning of African humanism, Mphahlele talks persuasively about the deep-seated belief of sub-Saharan Africans in the wisdom of the elders and the company of the ancestors. He also remarks on and encourages the tradition of the burial of the afterbirth or placenta by the mother or a close relative in the family compound, as a symbol of the circularity of the lifecycle, where the placenta represents a unique conjunction of the unborn, the born, and the ancestors as a tribute in the very ritual of burial. Mphahlele also addresses embodiment through the buried afterbirth, a metonymical part of the co-constituted effluent subject, unborn-living-ancestors-earth.

However, the very relation between African and European humanism is set in tension by the remarks with which Mphahlele reflects upon the importance of the tradition of the afterbirth.

One can perhaps see the "addition" of the ancestors to the notion of enduring humanism as that which makes (Mphahlele's) humanism African; but to do so would be simplistic in implying that all one needs for an African humanism is the substitution of African ontologies of being for Enlightenment (human) intelligence or epistemology. What Mphahlele says in detail is this:

> I should also say that in African humanism there is no dichotomy between the material world and the spiritual world. There is a continuity reinforced by interrelationships and interconnectedness. That is animal life, plant life and inanimate objects have a life of their own which is part of us. (Samin 1997, 184)

What Mphahlele then goes on to describe can be termed rituals, but only in the sense in which ritual is understood as a set of practices that dramatize the interrelatedness of inanimate materials, nature (animal and plant life), and human animals themselves. These rituals are not acts fixed in the nonending and nonchanging time of the Hegelian other that is the African subject of pre-1960s anthropology. Rather, "[when] a traditional healer will use organic matter to heal the body, it will be something plucked from nature, because there is a unity. Part of the continuity is also dramatized by the way in which women will take their afterbirth and bury it in the vicinity because it symbolizes reincarnation, the cyclical pattern of existence" (184).

One could see in Mphahlele's African humanism a kind of survivalist anthropocentrism with an African twist, that twist being the emphatically not (European) Christian reincarnation and/or the specifically not Western continuity between the unborn, the living, and the ancestors. However, this would be to overlook the important point at which Mphahlele sounds like a cross between a definitively European new materialist and a posthumanist: "Animal life, plant life, and inanimate objects have a life of their own which is part of us" (184).

The conflict between the term *inanimate* objects and the phrase "have a *life* of their own" (emphasis added) speaks precisely to that which cannot be spoken in English without making the language work against its historical episteme. In the same interview, Mphahlele expresses a desire to write a novel tentatively entitled *And the Birds Flew Away*, about two feuding neighbors and the weaver birds who live in the vicinity: "The weaver birds have a typical mythology, indifferent but almost as if they were aware of what is happening, of the conflict. But one winter time, shall I say one Autumn time, they take off, they're gone" (Samin 1997, 197).[16] Mphahlele is at pains to point out this is *not* some pathetic fallacy, some projection onto nature by the human intellect. "What bothers me here is, how can I convince anybody that this is not the intellect projecting itself into a situation where the relationship between animal life and African life, or human life, shall I say, is thus interwoven?" (198).

It is not accidental that Mphahlele sees the task of convincing others of this interwovenness highly challenging in the immediate wake of apartheid and before the attention had duly been paid to Indigenous knowledge systems in South Africa as valid in their own right, beyond the anthropologizing gaze of the colonizer and not as ever counterproductive to "Black health." An analogous task is taken up with vigor in Robin Wall Kimmerer's 2014 *Braiding Sweetgrass* and exemplified in Warren Cariou's 2018 "Sweetgrass Stories: Listening for Animate Land." But before we get to a place where, as Kimmerer puts it, we can imagine a world in which "people and land are good medicine for one another" (2014, x), we need to attend to the decolonial matter, by which I mean the work needed for us to be able to read the decolonizing stories that form the contours of Kimmerer's world, work in which this current chapter, and indeed this book as a whole, places itself.

There is a strain of melancholy in Mphahlele's work, as Samin highlights to Mphahlele himself. But this strain of melancholy is not because the birds fly away, if one may build on Mphahlele's prospective narrative, but because the birds that fly away are no longer able to do anything but witness human experience, as humans have lost the ability to be in relationship with the birds through the imposition of capitalist modernity: "They [the weaver birds] are now indifferent to human behavior whereas in earlier days we were all interlinked, we had a sense of interconnectedness with animal life" (198). If there is grievability here—and I argue there is—it is not about the migration of the weaver birds (which is in any event cyclical), but the loss of an African-humanist capacity to be in relation with the weaver birds. Understanding the impact of Cartesianism in its colonially imposed power is part of this work.

The need for this excess or effluence as that which is unspeakable to indeed *be spoken* (in English) is perhaps the root cause of melancholy in Mphahlele's work.[17] While Garuba has argued for materialist animism as a metaphorical ability of several literatures, including the work of Soyinka as a primary example, to express what I would call the animist element of effluence, I do not think Garuba's materialist animism "fixes" Mphahlele's conundrum. I argue, with Karen Barad (2003), that Mphahlele's melancholy rests on the post-Cartesian inability of English in practice to render "matter" and "spirit" simultaneous. It is also to be noted, as Kim (2015) has done, that, in the formulation of "matter" and "spirit," it is the Black body in particular that comes to represent the denigrated "matter" as opposed to the lofty "spirit" of the (white) human. English is not a neutral medium in which the Cartesian imaginary and the effluent imaginary meet on equal terms. Effluence provides a pathway for grieving what Cartesianism regards as waste, in which grief becomes an affirmation of the effluent subjects.

The emphasis Mphahlele puts on the burial of the afterbirth is probed by Samin in the question, not flippant, of what happens to the tradition of burying the placenta in the compound when one is no longer in the rural areas, but in the city. Mphahlele responds that he negatively sees the interruption of the tradition of midwifery and burial of the afterbirth in the modernization that leads to women giving birth in clinics and hospitals. After discussing the demise of this tradition, he comments that "African humanism has been battered a lot and we need to regain our balance" (Samin 1997, 184). Despite the nostalgic tone of this sentiment, the focus on the burial of the afterbirth, with its insistence on the inevitability of death and notion of the appropriate place for the ancestors as being with the material of the earth, seems to offer the linchpin I noted earlier: the key to comprehending the grievability of the human effluence, or how human effluence "it"self need not be grieved into chronic melancholy if it is attended to appropriately. Mphahlele suggests that grief is attended to appropriately if the rituals that maintain proper relations between the unborn, the living, and the ancestors are both properly undertaken and understood. How is this to be done in the specific context of the grievability we face less than a decade after Samin's interview with Mphahlele, that which accompanies the HIV/AIDS epidemic in sub-Saharan Africa?

What would a respectful yet nonanthropocentric, or animist, approach to grieving the effluent body-in-community of the HIV-sufferer look like? What kind of interconnection between inanimate material, animal life, and plant life may be entailed in grieving HIV-related death in the sub-Saharan African context that includes, but is not *confined* to, the HIV "victim" as the citizen who bears the right to HAART and related human rights? What or who is the subject in excess of their rights? How do we grieve the effluent subject? One can ask these questions without jumping to the notion that these deaths are of subjects without claims to rights. In that case, the deaths would be seen as "natural" or inevitable, and thus ungrievable in Butlerian terms. In the case of African AIDS, this approach justifiably invokes accusations of racism and resurrects the category of "African" as one of appropriate *un*grievability in the sense of Hegelian racism.[18]

The AIDS epidemic raises the question of how we might locate grievability in the face of overwhelming death, where such grievability does not depend on state recognition for the "legitimacy" of subjects of which the state may not know and about which it does not care, and where there may not be relatives to grieve the dead, owing to family separations under the pressures of postapartheid South Africa. As J. M. Coetzee's narrator puts it in *Diary of a Bad Year*, "Whether the citizen lives or dies is not a concern of the state. What matters to the state and its records is whether the citizen is alive or dead" (2007, 5). Further, family breakdown is so ubiquitous in rural parts of the country that there may not even be a family to grieve the dead, although I am not claiming by any means that this is always the case. But it is sufficiently common that its possibility needs to be reckoned with.

Grieving an Effluent Community: The AIDS-and-Daylily and Chicken-Suffering-Dying-and-Dead as Co-Constitutive Subject

In July 2004, the eThekwini (Durban metropolitan area) cemeteries department determined it would need an additional twelve hectares each year to accommodate the increased burial rate driven by the HIV epidemic. Of particular concern was identifying land in KwaMashu and Umlazi, where the majority of residents live and die. In 2013, the competition between land for development and land for burial became acute. Thembinkosi Ngcobo, head of eThekwini Parks, Recreation, and Culture Amenities, stated at the South African Cemeteries Association conference that land used for burial cannot legally be used for anything else and that burial grounds cannot be established within fifty meters of water sources, and the appropriate infrastructure has to be built according to environmental assessments (Mbonambi 2013).

Despite Gauteng having the largest population in South Africa, in 2010 the registered deaths in KwaZulu-Natal (KZN) exceeded those in Gauteng, with the largest number of deaths taking place in eThekwini (Mbonambi 2013). From 2003 to 2011, burial numbers in Durban appeared to gradually decline, but in 2013 the municipal cemeteries manager, Pepe Dass, pointed out that numerous staff had been dismissed for authorizing burials and then pocketing the money (Mbonambi 2013). Because of the respect for the dead and the traditional demands of the living to take care of ancestors' graves in relationships of mutual protection, the majority of the population of KZN do not view cremation as acceptable. In the case of unapproved and inappropriate burial sites, as well as inappropriate coffin materials, bodily fluids escape the grave and contaminate water sources. In 2010, the East Newlands burial ground became such a heavy source of coffin flies that it was later closed down, after heavier use of pesticides and other measures failed to control the proliferation of these flies in the surrounding neighborhood (Mbonambi 2013).[19]

In 2015, eThekwini announced that, if leases on graves were not renewed after ten years, those graves would be reused. Most religious leaders responded with horror, but the head of the cemeteries department for eThekwini argued that the practice could not be entirely new, as 1.5 million bodies are currently buried in approximately half a million graves in sixty-five cemeteries in the municipality. Arguably the most vociferous of the objections came from the KZN House of Traditional Leaders chair, then Inkosi Phathisizwe Chiliza, arguing that isiZulu culture does not allow the practice:

> In our culture, we respect graves. Once a person has passed away, we respect that person and we can't do anything to remove the grave except to discuss with the family. . . . If my father died today, even in 10 years, I will go and pay respects to my father at his grave and even my child will go there to respect his grandfather. If you bury someone over my father, what is that? (Comins 2015)

Rural areas are no less under pressure. In 2005, farm dwellers living on white-owned farms in KZN received the right to be buried on those farms. There had been tension over this issue, as such burials were believed by farm owners to prove subsequent support for land claims of farm dwellers against farm owners, and local authorities had frequently prevented such burials. Most rural burials take place in the family compounds.

However, the concern about appropriate burial as it is framed by the Enkosi amaKosi, or Chief of Chiefs, assumes that there is always a family to grieve the dead. But this is not always the case. From 2003 to 2013, I did field research and intervention work on a regular basis at St Apollinaris Hospital, Centocow, a district hospital of 155 beds about twenty minutes from the white farming settlement of Creighton. On one occasion, as we were giving a workshop on gender rights under the Constitution to hospital workers, my peripheral vision was often disturbed by what I would a second later recognize as gurneys coming down the open-air cement ramps from the upper floor of the hospital. These gurneys had bodies on them, many of them being taken to the incinerator, which was the case if the bodies were not claimed for burial. During the hour and a half of our workshop, about twelve bodies were taken out in this manner. The ramp became known to us colloquially, on the project, as Cadaver Way. We did not mean disrespect. We were trying to find words for such prevalence of death.

One day I was asked to meet with a young girl whose mother had just died. The mother had AIDS and was co-infected with (other) sexually transmitted infections. She left behind a daughter, whom I guessed, taking malnutrition into account, to be anywhere between eight and eleven, although I cannot of course be sure. The nurses were very embarrassed by the girl's behavior. After her mother died, she kept on flipping up her skirt to strangers in the hospital on the ward, and she had no underwear. They told me they had no idea of "what to do with her" until care was found, in the form of an orphanage willing to take her. Nursing is a highly respected and respectable profession, and in the rural areas it enables women to live away from men, in the nursing quarters attached to the hostels. In this context, the nurses were expressing the strangeness of the girl's behavior in their eyes, although having worked with abused children, I did not find her actions inexplicable. They were also overwhelmed by taking care of the sick, and this orphan was not visibly sick but certainly troubling to them. I explained to them that, in my view, she was seeking attention in the wake of her mother's death as best she knew how, which is why the nurses telling her to stop lifting her skirt was not working. I also convinced them that the most urgent act was not to find her underwear, but to engage her in a task with a nursing assistant or another patient, fold-ing linen or making beds, but at any event to keep her focused on a task with a companion. At this point I was completely focused on the challenge of respectful support of the girl myself, and not at all concerned about my own coherence in the scenario. I had not yet addressed the question of how I stood as a griever in relation to effluent subjects such as this girl, who had no one to grieve for and with her, as a newly orphaned child whose very behavior was perplexing to her current caregivers.

Later that day, I stumbled down the hill between St Appolinaris Hospital and the Centocow mission and was faced with a compound outside of which a chicken was tied up in forty-degree (Celsius) heat, obviously on hand to be slaughtered in the next few days, as it was Christmas week. The chicken was dying of heat exposure. I had no energy, nor the appropriate authority, nor the right as a privileged person with access to meat all year round if I wanted it, to do anything for the chicken, but I sat down and cried inconsolably in the land-cruiser, in the back seat, with my head down so no-one would see me. I have no idea how long I was there, nor did I know what I was crying *for*—a subject that in retrospect I identify as the effluent community of mother-orphan(with no relatives)-dying-daylily. Then I got up, let in a number of women seeking a lift to the closest transport stop on my way to Ixopo, and drove back to the project digs.

Once I saw Father Ignatius in a similar state. Father Ignatius is the priest at the Centocow mission, who attends every death at the hospital that he can, regardless of patients' religious affiliations, teaches the community boys football, and soothes his soul by growing daylilies just outside the mission, in the most extraordinary burst of colors ever found in the Centocow valley. (He used to "do" orchids, but these proved too difficult to tend in the climate of the Sisonke/Harry Gwala District.) *Hemerocallis* is called "daylily" because each bloom lasts only a day. Each scape (a stem that itself yearly grows and dies back) carries many blooms that open in succession, but each bloom itself is a one-day wonder. Father Ignatius was just a few months away from his sabbatical in his native Poland but was collapsing in view of this "finishing line." I sat as he told me a number of broken-up stories, all about how deaths had ravaged through the families he knew and did not know. He kept repeating that these were all "good people." He could not stop weeping from the most enormous set of blue eyes I have ever seen. (Ignatius is tall and thin and has dark hair, which makes the blue eyes even more dominant on his visage than would otherwise be the case).

I listened until he had no more energy to talk. We sat looking at the daylilies for a while, and they looked back at us. Then we went our separate ways, back to what I call coping life, which is not quite the same as coping with life.

Father Ignatius Stankiewicz, now returned from his sabbatical, is still at the Centocow Mission, which celebrated its 125-year jubilee in 2020.

When anyone asks me about the hardest moments of those years, before the widespread rollout of HAART and its beneficial effects were anywhere in evidence, I am embarrassed to say I just shake my head and change topics. How do you explain that your worst moment was when a chicken was dying of dehydration in a Christmas compound, or when a frog snuck into your computer bag at night to keep warm and you didn't know and the next day they were the soft squish you put your computer onto and you couldn't stop grieving?

The clinical way of explaining this, as I know perfectly well, is that the nonhuman animals' suffering is a trigger for the grief of all the dying and suffering and human deaths witnessed. True. But I don't think that's all there is to it.

If the bodies of the human animals and the bodies of the chicken (yet to die) and the frog (already dead) and the orphan inspire grievability in me, this is certainly not a grievability the South African state would countenance, nor yet empathize with. That African bodies have been too long rendered as mere animals would be a predictable response. Why would you dream of repeating the racist paradigm of the Black body as patently nonhuman and animal instead? A correlative response would be: Why would you pathologize the otherness of the HIV-positive Black body through its association with animalization?

The problem here is that the primary identity of these beings does not, in African humanism, depend on the binary alive–dead. Indeed, many of us who worked in and through the height of the epidemic prior to widespread HAART rollout developed an intimacy with the almost dead and dead bodies, such that our grief was not dependent on whether, or did not change if, the person was visibly dying or dead, a he, a she, a they, or an "it."

Once I was in Ixopo with a colleague to visit the district health officer. We were waiting in the land-cruiser until the December thunderstorm let up a bit. We saw two men get out of a tiny *bakkie,* one of those Hyundai trucks that looks like it just came out of a matchbox. They seemed to be carrying something very slight between them, like a sheet or a blanket, something very two-dimensional, and almost as tall as they were, but not quite. It wasn't glass because they were lined up in parallel: a man, the thing, and another man, with this narrow thing between them.

Once they came a meter or two closer we realized it was a very sick man between them. So sick, in fact, that he was barely there, like a slip of a man: one slip and you wouldn't have known he had been there. We sat shocked to the core that there could be so little difference between the barely living and the dead.

Later, we became more used to this weird fact, that near-deathness or death made no difference to the grief. It just felt slightly, I don't know, *sacred* maybe, to witness a being between death and life and then also a being between death and whatever that death means to the being that is dead, in the process of becoming-ancestor. Mother, chicken, frog, even daylily—they were becoming different, ancestors bearing witness to us, we who were flailing about trying to cope-live. We thought we were bearing witness to them, but somehow, each time, they seemed to be grieving for our inability to make our joy and our grief adequate to *their* being. We were always struggling to exceed our own grief to pay them the respect they properly commanded. Our grief was "all about us."

So I began to think about these effluent bodies (unclaimed humans, almost dead chicken, dead frog, daylily dying on its one day of glory) not as subjects for the elegy, but as subjects in excess of their rights: in excess of the rights of the human to full citizenship, antiretrovirals; in excess of humans as victims of "failing social and economic networks of support . . . becom[ing] differentially exposed to injury, violence, and death" (Butler 2009, 25); the frog as one whom one should not mourn as much as the human; the chicken as continuously disposable, the daylily as built for what we might call natural disposability. What, Mphahlele might ask us, can we hear these beings saying? Can we listen? Can grievability be a listening? Can grievability be anything other than a bearing witness? Is there a way of modeling effluent grief when there are no families to undertake extra-anthropocentric rituals?

Firstly, many of the people who(se bodies) remained unclaimed at Centocow were always living without networks of social and economic support due to the apartheid and postapartheid family breakdown I was talking about earlier. One can think about this as people living in the cracks the state leaves open in a metaphorical road, only in rural KZN there are more cracks than there are roads, metaphorical and literal; and family erosion and poverty during and after apartheid make these cracks intergenerational. Further, these effluent bodies prove that the recognizable grievability of the state or the person, as conceived of in Butler's formulation, may capture the experience of grievability from an anthropocentric viewpoint, but not from the perspective of what we might call a latter-day African humanist, a descendant of Mphahlele's narrative. For, what is the unborn but precisely something that is most categorically of life, just as that which is dead is not "not of life," but an ancestor?

When Stephanie Nolen was completing her 2008 *28 Stories of AIDS*, she asked me what the center was of the crisis that the sub-Saharan epidemic had precipitated. I explained that one could describe it in Stephen Lewis-like terms:[20] that grannies were being forced to raise young children, that men and women of income-earning age were dying, that the South African state under President Thabo Mbeki[21] seemed impervious to the HIV/AIDS epidemic, but what was one to do if people were dying before they had enough experience to become ancestors to the living? This seems to me to be the cosmological crux of the grief of the epidemic: the inconsolable grief of the living that the dead might not become ancestors, or adequate ancestors, owing to their youth. What we could be being asked to hear from these unauthorized ancestors in graves from East Newlands, to the compounds of KZN, to the dead frogs and flowers in garbage heaps and to the incinerated is *not* to stop demanding rights, but to assume that human rightness might be reconceived from the perspective of the dead, because orthodox human rights assume that death has no subjectivity. A correlative of the dead-have-no-subjectivity assumption is that the effluent body (leaking waste or dead, and therefore becoming waste) cannot be grieved, and therefore cannot be thought to have lived.

But the effluent body speaks. Sometimes it yells through the unseemliness of its effluence, as when "it" pushes away a computer from its absurd frog-ly dignity, or brings down a plague of coffin flies on those who look to ignore "it," or permeates the air of the valley with the smell of burning flesh from the incinerator, or resounds with its claims to beauty on the day of "its" "death," with human and nonhuman animal "death" all around "it," like the daylily. If we don't listen, that's not yet another responsibility of the effluent being.

It's ours.

And in relinquishing such listening, we give up material forms of persistence; we give up whole realms of desire that can and do resist their condemnation as effluent, toxic, a kind of metonymical necrophilia—indeed, waste and waste of time. Mourning, desire, and beauty are the language in which the desired and desiring "dead" speak to us. This is not an exotic call to action, but a quotidian exchange of extra-anthropocentric beings, and the rightness of such being. Its value is unspeakable within the current genre of the "human," but lies in the imaginative reordering of human rightness that would render conventional genres of the human and their constructions of disposability not only visible as profoundly wasteful, but indeed as toxic to nonanthropocentric human rightness.

2

Effluence in Disease

Ebola and HIV as Case Studies of Debility in the Postcolonial State

Key to the vision of rights deployed in the United Nations 1948 *Declaration of Human Rights* (UNDHR) is the right to "the highest attainable standard of health as a fundamental right of every human being," as I noted in the introduction. The state is central to the UNHR project, just as the state is central, paradoxically in its absence, to Judith Butler's formulation of grievability. The World Health Organization (WHO) claims:

> Understanding health as a human right creates a legal obligation on states to ensure access to timely, acceptable, and affordable health care of appropriate quality as well as to providing for the underlying determinants of health, such as safe and potable water, sanitation, food, housing, health-related information and education, and gender equality. (WHO 2017b)[1]

There are primarily two players in this version of rights: the state, as provider, and the citizen, as entitled to the right to health. There is an acknowledgment, however, of the diminishment of some states' role in the provision of healthcare in the face of Big Pharma. WHO observes that:

> States and other duty-bearers are answerable for the observance of human rights. However, there is also a growing movement recognising the importance of other non-state actors such as businesses in the respect and protection of human rights. (WHO 2017b)

In this aspirational rhetoric, we see that such rights are inalienable but at the same time need to be achieved, as is the case with Hannah Arendt's subject-in-need-of-rights who cannot claim them because He does not command them already. We can also recognize that the very building block of these rights, the citizen, is fully within the Sylvia Wynter's "genre of man." Defenders of the rights regime of health argue that the WHO pays specific attention to gender, Indigenous health, HIV-positive subjects, and other "conditions" of being they regard as potentially detrimental to the principle of nondiscrimination:

> Any discrimination, for example in access to health care, as well as in means and entitlements for achieving this access, is prohibited on the basis of race, color, sex, language, religion, political or other opinion, national or social origin, property, birth, physical or mental disability, health status (including HIV/AIDS), sexual orientation, and civil, political, social or other status, which has the intention or effect of impairing the equal enjoyment or exercise of the right to health. (WHO, 2017)

Here we have a beneficiary who is not only assumed to be a citizen, or at the very least has access to a "state or other duty-bearer" to whom He can appeal for health. He is also assumed to occupy a naturalized state of healthiness. Normally it is assumed that the passage's attention to various situations in respect of which there should be no discrimination includes subject-citizens who may exhibit characteristics that bring down discrimination on them, inhibiting their access to health. On the contrary, I argue, not only do such formulations resurrect the implicit subject as identical to Wynter's genre of the human, but they also imply He is the epitome of the healthy. Gender, sexual orientation, HIV status, and so on—in fact, all "conditions" denied or not represented by the genre of man are liberal exceptions that must be "added on" to the genre of man to be subsequently recognized in order to create a nondiscriminatory environment for access to health. This is an ableist approach to disease. The effluent eye offers a rendering of the subject as perpetually a subject in conditions that produce debility, rather than modeling the putative healthy citizen in the first instance.

In this chapter, I look at colonialism in relation to health as an example of a condition that is not mentioned in the rights to health documents of the UNDHR, that is intergenerational in its effects, and that counters the personalization of negative affect attached to an individual identity, such as race or age. I pull back from the immediacy of the effluent deaths I grieved and attempted to honor at the conclusion of the last chapter to focus more broadly on the relations between effluence and debility, using colonialism as the medium in which these exist. I ask how one might develop a truly decolonial methodology of writing medical history. I instantiate debility as the norm of effluent communities, outside of the extreme conceptualizations of disability as exceptional and ability as normal. I look at what are currently called the social and economic "determinants" of health critically, meaning in terms of their inadequacy for effluent formulations, which take into account colonial capitalism as a violent structural constraint. To state the point in a different way, the effluent eye does not envision that there is a norm (the "human" of the UNDHR, of the genre of man) onto which debility is attached after the fact of Him. That is to say, "race," national origin, and the power structures in which they are imbricated are intersectional realities at the very origins of the human. What's more, fear of disease more often than not plays out in contexts of colonialist-capitalist legacy, in which health is seen as a service, not a common good; where individuals and states still seek to attach blame to global flows of disease, instead of understanding disease as what I call a companion of humanity, evolving concomitantly between humans and nonhuman animals; and where stigma is attached indelibly to disease and debilitated bodies precisely because such bodies are not human. They are not healthy, are not productive, have a threatened ability to consume goods, and do not fall within the genre of man. Our ability to speak the commonness of debility, however, is very much under censorship, to the extent that colonial capitalism depends on debilitated workers (slaves, colonized peoples, indentured laborers, migrant laborers in poor working conditions) for its productivity, just as much as such productivity produces a debilitated earth and companion animals in its wake.

I focus primarily on Ebola (in West Africa) and HIV (in sub-Saharan Africa) as examples of colonially engendered diseases. Both, like Covid-19, are zoonoses, diseases that have jumped the species barrier from nonhuman animals to human animals; and both, again like Covid-19, have to do with increasingly closer communion between animals and nonhuman animals because of human movements. Ebola has its origins in areas where deforestation has occurred at rapid rates, displacing nonhuman animals into areas of higher human traffic, in the Ebola River region in northern Democratic Republic of Congo (DRC). Reuse of needles at the local missionary hospital escalated the spread in the first outbreak in 1976. HIV has its origins in the Kinshasa region of the same country, between 1910 and 1930, when the virus jumped the species boundary from its simian origin, initially probably as a consequence of bush hunting. What drove its spread, however, was the rapid growth of Leopoldville, the former name of Kinshasa, which was the capital of what later became the Belgian Congo.

I am not suggesting that, without colonialism, there would be no disease. I am saying that to consider the social determinants of health outside of the complex histories of colonialism is absurd, much like trying to ascertain the shape of an object through two dimensions only, and further, that to ignore the neocolonialism of Western medicine is not only unethical, but runs against its own historical mandate: "First, do no harm." Let us turn our attention to the era of the contemporary millennium and see how colonial capitalism is both unspeakable as a social and economic determinant of health and yet crucial to understanding the history of the diseases in question.

Ebola and HIV Narratives in a Colonialist-Capitalist World

In October 2014, Ebola costumes sold out for Halloween. There was the Ebola HAZMAT costume (modeled by a boy in the ads), and two versions of the "sexy Ebola containment suit" (girl's costume, designed to show leg at the risk of compromising the fiction of its containment properties). Many felt this was "in bad taste," as Arthur Kaplan, head of the bioethics division at New York University's Langone Medical Center, put it (cited in Baskas 2014). Doctors of the World, a humanitarian organization, used the opportunity to advertise for donations of protective equipment to be used in the affected countries of Guinea, Sierra Leone, and Liberia, deploying a campaign entitled "It's more than a Halloween costume" with the accompanying tagline, "Here it's a Costume; There it saves Lives" (Baskas 2014). In Sacramento, Robert Kirk, a therapist at Sage Psychotherapy, said making a serious situation seem humorous could be viewed in the light of a defense mechanism; people play up the issue to keep genuinely fear-generating situations "at arm's length, kind of a whistling-past-the-graveyard kind of thing" (cited in Caiola 2014). Why, one might ask, would Americans be so fearful of Ebola?

Contemporaneous news articles claimed President Barack Obama's affinity with Africa through his grandfather's Kenyan origins meant that he was prepared to sacrifice American security by refusing to cut off the United States from West African air traffic during the epidemic. Dr. Keith Ablow, of the Fox News's "Medical A-Team," claimed that Obama's "affinities" are with Africa, not the United States: "His affinities, his affiliations are with them, not us. . . . He's their leader." Ablow elaborated on what he sees as Obama's perspective:

> In his mind, if only unconsciously, he's thinking, "Really? We're going to prevent folks suffering with illnesses from coming across the border flying into our airports when we have visited a plague of colonialism that has devastated much of the world, on the world? What is the fairness in that?" How can you protect a country you don't like? Why would you? (cited in Hananoki 2014)

This tells us more about Ablow's fears and preoccupations than about Obama's; and those are not singular to Ablow. Radio host Rush Limbaugh suggested Obama refused to divert flights from Ebola-infected countries and close down America's borders because Obama believed the United States "deserves" to be infected with Ebola as retribution for its role in perpetuating slavery (cited in Volsky 2014).

Responding to a caller on his nationally syndicated radio show, Limbaugh launched into a soliloquy: ". . . [the United States] being to blame for things and it's that kind of thinking that leads to opposition to shutting down airports from various countries," he explained, referring to the Obama administration's handling of the crisis. "It leads to opposition to keeping these people out of the country: 'How dare we? We can't turn our back on them! They exist because of us. We can't turn them away!'" (cited in Volsky 2014). Limbaugh vocalizes his notion of politically correct liberals, whom he thinks believe that the United States is responsible for the spread of Ebola in Liberia because that nation was established by freed American slaves. "And if it hadn't been for that they probably wouldn't have [Ebola]. So there are some people who think we kind of deserve a little bit of this," he said, before accusing American leaders of purposely leaving the U.S. vulnerable to the virus: "The danger we have now is that we elected people in positions of power and authority who think this or think like this in terms of this country being responsible" (cited in Volsky 2014).

While some may have dismissed Ablow and Limbaugh, both associated with the Fox News network, as extremist voices, what is striking about the Ebola outbreak of 2014 is the complex set of affects attending on its coverage in the Unites States. These cannot be assigned to mere bad taste or what was, before Trump's election, often described as marginal politics. Such affects include fear of, and fascination with, a nationally conceived power that can ostensibly "save" and "kill"—the kind of biopolitics Giorgio Agamben associates with a sovereign (1998). This amounts to a fetishization of a political power, conceptually aligned with the nation-state, to foster life or disallow it to the point of death, or as Achille Mbembe puts it, revisiting Foucault, involved in "the generalized instrumentalization of human existence and the material destruction of human bodies and populations" (2003, 14). Here I am using the definition of the fetish as an object that is always fantastical to the extent it substitutes for another object or condition perceived to be missing (Suleiman 1990, 48).

This fascination with a (putative) sovereign power is expressed in the Halloween costumes, as well as in rants against Obama as refusing to protect the United States because of his affiliation with African-ness, in a specifically biomedical iteration. This affiliation marks Obama as incapable as a Black man, despite his U.S. citizenship, of exercising that citizenship in favor of U.S. citizens, in an old equation in which Blacks cannot be sufficiently American; but simultaneously, the president of the United States should let Africans die ostensibly to save U.S. citizens. Here Obama is attributed with believing that Ebola marks a retributive justice for the exercise of the slave trade by white Americans against nonwhite ones; and responsibility for Liberians, as citizens of the U.S.-initiated exslave colony, is seen as the revenant of the duties owed to Liberia by those U.S. authorities who literally made the state (possible) in the first instance. Obama is the "object" who is inadequate as fetish because he cannot represent the subjective power of a white president.

Juxtapose this scene with one almost a decade earlier, in 2003, when I was interviewing inhabitants of the Sisonke/Harry Gwala District of KwaZulu-Natal (KZN) about their ideas of how HIV came to be so pervasive in the region, most of which is deeply rural and not easy to access. An older lady in the Underberg area told me that the apartheid government had inflicted HIV on Blacks in South Africa in retribution for the Black majority voting for the African National Congress (ANC) in 1994, which led to the election of the first postapartheid government under Nelson Mandela. A response to such a statement might have been to dismiss her as ignorant. However, this lady spoke a certain truth. The apartheid government was extremely slow to acknowledge and deal with HIV/AIDS while simultaneously ordering HIV-positive agents to infiltrate ANC cadres and infect them. Further, the government funded a program to develop strains of bacteria and viruses that would target the Black population, a project that was predictably a failure, as race is not a category that works in terms of infectious disease perpetration. Sterilization of Black women and HIV-positive women without their consent has been documented in South Africa and Namibia, although racially motivated programs involving disease agents cannot be made to target one race over another.

The lady had an embodied, intergenerational knowledge of apartheid biopolitics and their racist aspirations. She would have had no problem comprehending the connections between racism and its effects in terms of structural violence, of the relative vulnerability of Black and Brown people in the United States to Covid-19. It would be a misrecognition to think of her and Ablow and Limbaugh as speaking with the same validity. Ablow and Limbaugh have not experienced a state deploying power against them in the form of racist provisions for separate education, job reservation, racially directed population control, and so on. Their sense of threat is precisely what makes their response to Ebola fantastical.

So how does the fantasy of the Ebola threat play out specifically along racial lines? The response to Ebola manifests a fantasy of containment of the (racialized) threat of exotic disease, wherein the costume acts as a staging of whites both as impervious to disease though proper technologies of protection and as "saving" Blacks, where the doctor/nurse is preconceived of as white, and the patient, missing from the costume but implied by it, is black African. The fact that the disease made it into a Halloween costume is related to the virtual impossibility of getting Ebola in the United Kingdom or America, where the costumes were bestsellers. The racial politics would have played out differently if that were the case. It's hard to believe a Covid-19-related costume would make it onto the shelves because it "lives" in the United States already, across Black, Brown, and white populations, although the former two groups are differentially negatively affected. Indeed, one of the reasons HIV in America has such a different cultural profile from Ebola is because it, too, "lives" in the United States and is distinguished from the sub-Saharan epidemic by the telling phrase "African AIDS." (There is, to my knowledge, no North American correlate, such as "American AIDS.") It is revealing that all the advertisements for the popular 2014 Ebola Halloween costume feature whites sporting their safeguards in various parodies of personal preventative equipment (PPE, the Centers for Disease Control [CDC] term that has become so familiar to us from news coverage of the U.S. response to Covid-19).

The fascination is with the epidermalized white fantasy of the power of healing, of saving from death, while oneself being immune. The unexpressed terror is that of becoming ill, becoming Black, becoming unruly through improper contact with the racialized other who manifests these supposedly negative attributes. One can think of the unspoken element of this fear in the fact that, as I noted above, there is no "pair" costume for the Ebola doctor or nurse. This would have been "for" the Ebola victim, just as there are numerous vampire-and-victim Halloween costume pairs. One could interpret this absence as politically correct, but that has certainly not been the case in other aspects of popular costumes, where fear of social sanction has been notably absent. Rather, the ellipsis of a partner Halloween figure expresses the "impossibility" of a white Ebola victim, even in play. The fantasy of immunity manifests itself in fear of contamination, which is itself not logical, where the figure of the diseased, racialized, and unrulable other threatens citizenry who are the apotheosis of the genre of the human and need to be maintained by a racialized *cordon sanitaire*. Americans too may "get sick" (contaminated), hence the need for a "wall," now translated into Trump's fantasy wall, that will protect Americans. Paranoia and racialized images of the diseased as disposable abound in the performance, rather than the actuality, of Ebola as an exotically constructed threat. These images portray the diseased as surplus to requirements, as that material set of objects (non-animated) that need to be contained. What cannot be contained in the white fantasy of immunity is a set of conjoined effluent subjects whose moniker would be something like Black-diseased-mad-unruly-unrulable-noncitizen, prefigured in the historical figure of the slave and suggested by the very idea of Ebola as a Halloween costume.

The cultural logic behind the adoption of the Ebola costume can be traced to the predominance of the zombie in Halloween costumes. The zombie, originating in Haitian folklore, represents a "walking dead" body, often thought to be contaminated by having been bitten by another zombie, since the zombie is a voracious, flesh-eating being with malevolent intent. The zombie most likely derived from transformations of West African folklore that originated in the seventeenth century when West African slaves were brought to work on the Haitian sugar plantations. The zombie is, in this context, thought to represent the miserable conditions under which slaves labored for their owners. The waking-dead aspect of this suggests the notion that one cannot escape slavery, even in death. However, I propose it also has a persistent meaning, or in the context of this argument, possibly an effluent one: the walking dead may wake at any moment to resist their incarceration, just as the ancestors may advise the living to rebel against structural violence, consisting in slavery, impoverishment, and illness at the behest of colonial capitalism, racist governance, and their intersection. The latter interpretation, it is worth noting, is possible only if one holds the cycle of the unborn, the living, and the ancestors as an ontology of relations that confound the normative Western binary of living–dead.

The constellation of images doing culturally violent work in the 2014 Ebola outbreak challenges us to compose a history of disease and human being coexistence that bears witness to effluent subjects who are pitted against the healthy genre of the human that inhabits the UNDHR. An effluent eye enables comprehension of the genre of the human as linking practices of colonialism and medicine through a shared politics. Both colonialism and medicine tend to see disease and the diseased subject as that which should be confined to objectivity, and consequently be ejected from the modern state or the individual respectively. This is the case despite the facts that constantly vulnerable and debilitated subjects are essential to the survival of the colonialist-capitalist contemporary state, through its dependence on exploitable labor, and that one cannot separate disease from its co-constitutive "host," or to paraphrase Yeats's words, in disease, one cannot know the dancer from the dance (see "Among School Children" in Yeats 1989, 64).

The first fact above (reliance on constantly debilitated and vulnerable subjects) constitutes the foundational contradiction of capitalism in this study: capitalism promises material benefits to all, but simultaneously depends upon exploitative labor practices and global inequity. Effluent subjects in this context are anti-utopian within the settler-state political imaginary, where utopianism acts as a racialized and "healthy" containment strategy. Effluence can and does dwell domestically; and the specter of the improper "citizen," or of citizens' contact with disallowed subjects, who are perceived as objects, is insupportable because it reminds the citizenry that effluent subjects are not confined to the exotic. This is spectacularly problematic, as only specialized cohorts of citizens "should" have contact with effluent subjects.

In the case of this chapter, the specialists are humanitarian global health physicians whose job it is explicitly to heal the vulnerable, but implicitly to "take the flak" to keep the citizenry at home safe, in a medical model that uses humanitarianism to feed exotic interest and to stage Western medicine as infinitely superior to Indigenous forms of healing within the postcolonial context. For this reason, I conclude with a critique of the utopianism/neocolonialism of the role of Western medicine in humanitarian interventions in the global South, and by rethinking the *figure of the zombie*, not as one who simply answers the capitalist call to work-for-money-and-purchase-goods as an end in and of itself, but as signaling the birth of *the as-yet-to-be-materialized possibility that productivity can be recognized outside of colonialist-capitalist frameworks*. First, however, I trace the histories of utopian attempts to keep out Blackness, to keep out diseases, as colonialist and neocolonialist operations that seek to deny both the fact of effluent subjects within state borders and these operations' dependence on slave labor and its descendent, an endlessly substitutable labor force. I conclude with a critique of the utopianism/neocolonialism of Western medical practices in interventions in the global South, and by rethinking the figure of the "duppy," or zombie, as that which simply answers the capitalist call to "work-for-money-and-purchase-goods" as an "ethic" and end in and of itself.[2]

The kind of vulnerability generated by the fear–aggression matrix evident in Ebola fantasies does not attach to the effluent subject, who lives alongside both the real possibility of and the actuality of illness. Where that illness is accompanied by conditions of colonialist-capitalist structural violence, effluent subjects find ways of naming that violence, as did the lady of rural KZN in her discussion with me. Determining responsibility at an individual rather than structural level is the challenge in naming structural violence in a context of ideological domination by the vocabulary of the genre of the human and its relation to the citizen; the vocabulary makes structural violence invisible as a determinant of health. Think, for example, of all the demonized individuals/nationalities associated with the spread of Covid-19 in the United States, as in "China flu." Invisible detrimental conditions are assignable to the effluent other in figures of unspeakability, as in the implied but missing partner Ebola costume. What xenophobic naming masks, however, is our connectedness to China through global networks and the fault lines that the virus illuminates domestically, within the United States. In the global postcolony, neither the technologies of Western medicine nor their power to save are untouched by such structural threat.

The term currently used by the National Institutes of Health (NIH) to describe contexts of health debility is the "social determinants of health" (SDH), sometimes expanded to the "social and economic determinants of health" (SEDH). According to the CDC, the term SDH "refers to the complex, integrated and overlapping social structures and economic systems that include the social physical environments and health services. These determinants are shaped by the level of income, power, and resources at global, national, and local levels . . . often influenced by policy choices" (2010).[3] The CDC and the NIH base their definition on the U.N. report finalized in 2008, conducted by the WHO Commission on Social Determinants of Health. Interestingly, the places where the term is most employed is in relation to explicitly recognized "vulnerable populations"; so, for example, the websites in which it plays a greater role than elsewhere in the NIH sites include the CDC's National Center for HIV/AIDS, Viral Hepatitis, STD, and TB Prevention and the National Institute of Minority Health and Health Disparities. This gives the unfortunate impression that the structural violence of inequity can best be addressed through attention to minority health concerns. Yet the absent partner in this picture is the idea of medicine as a key site of corporate profit. Attention is paid to victims of structural violence, but not to its beneficiaries in financial terms, or to intergenerational histories that produce such negative outcomes.

It should come as no surprise, then, that an analogous problem affects the history of relations between settler-colonial enterprises and disease, especially infectious disease, where colonially directed population movements are left out of medical history. In 1998, Warwick Anderson wrote a review of two histories—on the developments of tropical medicine and of colonial medicine in Malaysia—tellingly entitled "Where Is the History of Postcolonial Medicine?," in which he argues that:

> Over the past twenty years or so, a small but growing band of historians of medicine has directed its attention to disease and health care in colonial settings. Previously, medicine and imperialism had been brought together mainly in the recollections of colonial medical officers and in the more wide-ranging social histories of

recently decolonized nations. In these accounts, Western medicine was generally presented as one of the few indubitable benefits of European imperialism. Even Frantz Fanon, the Martiniquean psychiatrist who features so prominently in origin stories of postcolonial critique, remained convinced that Western medicine and psychiatry were basically good things, although distorted in a colonial structure of inequalities. But historians of colonial medicine are now more likely to discern a deeper collusion between medicine and empire: the political economists among them describe more plausibly a colonial production of disease, and the more literary of them analyze medicine and public health as technical discourses of colonialism. Accordingly, it seems now that to use Western methods to prevent or treat the diseases spread by colonialism was to colonize the body in a more basic way than Fanon's nationalist optimism would ever let him admit.

So have we, then, developed a truly postcolonial historiography of Western medicine, our own postcolonial literature? I do not think so. Rather, it seems to me that we are successfully building a disciplinary enclave of implicitly nationalist historians of medicine. We are more likely to ask what is distinctive about Western medicine in a particular colonial, or protonational, setting than to look for what is colonial about Western medicine in any setting. We are still writing a minor literature. (522–23)

To take up Anderson's challenge, I look for what might be colonial about Western medicine through an explicitly *non*nationalist history involving Ebola and HIV/AIDS. These diseases, as I noted earlier, are thought of within nationalist imaginaries as African, where "Africa" is not (even) yet acknowledged to have states, even though those states were in the first instance determined by Europeans at the 1885 Berlin Conference. First, I connect the concept of the state-as-healthy to the human subject, to illustrate the ubiquity of the genre of the "healthy human" subject in its enmeshment in practices of human-rights violations through colonization and slavery and through the instrumentalization of some human beings. I associate this with an essentially vulnerable utopianism, one whose weakness lies in its addiction to the state-as-healthy and its projection of the unhealthy onto noncitizens who are then cast as enemies, standing in for the oft-imagined danger of "the" (usually "an," meaning the handiest politically at the time) infectious disease with pandemic "street cred," the infectious disease that's trending, one might say. When I have demonstrated the challenge the elision of nonnationalist, postcolonial histories of medicine[4] poses to rendering structural violence in terms of SEDH, I move, albeit tentatively, toward explication of an effluent subject: an explication that distinguishes between biological disease agents and the structural violence that enables them to flourish.

I embark on a brief, comparative history of the heavily burdened postcolonies of Liberia, Sierra Leone, and Haiti to begin filling the gap Warwick has outlined. While recent feminist thought has begun to understand that autonomy must, of necessity, entail vulnerability in terms of constructive interdependence, I describe forms of sovereignty that seek to deny vulnerability in fantasies of absolute domination at the very birth of nation-states.[5] That is to say, I identify within the very ideation of the nation-state a utopian will to power that is mystified by the independent agency of potentially damaging but entirely nonintentional forms of threat to state governance, such as is the paradigmatic case in this chapter, infectious disease. I pay particular attention to the material realities of the ebbs and flows, crossings and recrossings, of trade in persons and diseases and their shared materiality, attempting to place this history of material exchanges within an understanding of settler-colonial and late-capitalist utopian dreams of sovereignty, where the utopia must, by definition, exclude any ideation of vulnerability. Unlike this utopian will to power, whose goal is an impossibly consistent invulnerability, the effluent subject accepts vulnerability as a condition of being, without the anthropocentric attribution of self-denial ("I am invulnerable") or masochism ("I am always a victim"). The acceptance of vulnerability as ontological is frequently interpreted in global capitalism as self-victimization (the "pull yourself up by your bootstraps" approach to structural violence). While one can attribute a politics to the intentionality of human forces driving population ebbs and flows in a colonial context, taking a decentered approach to the agency of disease involves entangling histories of human intentionality in a new sociality with histories of disease, while scrupulously avoiding assigning agency to diseases such as AIDS and Ebola outside of their hardwiring to reproduce and thrive at the material level. This kind of history begins to answer Anderson's call for postcolonial medical history through a decolonial critique. The vexed question of how to write postcolonial medical history with decolonial vision requires writing medical history outside of the genre of the anthropocentric human, portrayed either as "savior" (the desire behind the Ebola containment suit) or "victim" (the absent and feared Ebola sufferer).

My refusal to assign agency to diseases outside of their biological hardwiring is not to deny that such diseases play a role in vast symbolic imaginaries of humans, such as those that locate AIDS as a sign of moral failure and Ebola as racialized proof of an inherent weakness or inability to thrive. Such inability precedes the onset of the disease and is made explicit by the disease, under the sign of impropriety, in which the disease becomes the outward manifestation of the mistake of improper, unapproved contact with effluent subjects. Such impropriety is true for the Black ~~subject~~object, as well as for that often unnervingly, indeterminate ~~subject~~object, the yet-to-be-out-as-HIV-positive person whose "preexisting condition" of disease masquerades as the healthy citizen.

It is, however, crucial to separate these imaginaries from an understanding of the agency of the diseases themselves, to "reverse engineer" disease history to see diseases as "companion animals," so to speak, to colonial and capitalist enterprises of accumulation through dispossession. I invoke companion animals in the same way in which Donna Haraway speaks of dogs as companion animals to humans in her 2003 *Companion Species Manifesto*. To paraphrase her key questions about dogs and humans (3) in terms of humans and viruses: How might an ethics and politics of significant otherness be learned from taking the human–disease agent relationships seriously? And how might stories about disease–human worlds finally convince Americans that history matters in naturecultures?[6] Here "naturecultures" is a description of an effluent subject that refuses to separate human-as-cultural from nonhuman-as-natural, or "primitive," resulting in the telltale conjoined subject that is impossible within the Enlightenment imaginary that separates (white) Human Subject from (Black) nonhuman object.

The bare facts of the history I reprise below concerning an array of transatlantic crossings, and indeed crosshatchings, involving the colonial management of (quasi) subjects (that is, colonially ruled peoples) are not new.[7] My contribution aims to contextualize these facts within a nexus of hyperimages of slavery, disease, "race," zombification, and nationalism around which the fear and fascination I referenced above in relation to the figure of the Ebola Halloween costume coalesce. These are hyperimages in the same way that Timothy Morton describes his "hyperobjects" as such enormously and variously inflected images that we have trouble tracing their implications comprehensively because we live within them, rather than look at them (2013). These implications escape articulation within the framework of individual or even collective human subjectivity and agency. That is to say, they are inarticulable within frameworks driven purely by the bildungsroman/human-rights aspiration of man-as-sovereign, His intentions and their consequences as controlled and effective, and the nation-state as the primary mechanism of communal expression of those intentions and their consequences.

The truths spoken by these hyperimages begin to become more visible only in a rendering of them in which sovereign/colonizing Man is visible in the center of a structural violence, colonial capitalism, that reflects the narcissism of an anthropocentric world.[8] The hyperimages, the expression of fused desire and terror that accompany sovereign fantasy, have identifiable historical roots and deeply important effects on current global biopolitics. Further, their entanglements extend into negative public-health outcomes. I frame these outcomes as the materialization of racist utopia/dystopia fantasies, characterized by their inability to face the vulnerability the supposedly nonhuman other (Black, African, slave, disease) presents to the human. In effect, I describe how the human that exceeds the normative intentionality attributed to Him in the genre of the human, manifest in the UNDHR, sets panic to work in the administrative heart of colonialist-capitalist "rationality," as evidenced in Ebola Halloween costumes explicated above.

Slavery as the Instantiation of Capital at the Founding of the Nation-State: Sierra Leone, Liberia, Haiti

The three countries most deeply affected by Ebola in 2014—Sierra Leone, Liberia, and Guinea—were profoundly influenced by precolonial and colonial slave trading. Specifically, Sierra Leone and Liberia were founded by freed slaves. That is to say, some white abolitionists and freed Black allies held the view that having slaves freed in the United Kingdom and the United States settle "back" in West Africa was ideal. These freed slaves were part of the intergenerational displacement of the slaves from Africa in the transatlantic slave-trade practices of forced removal and abduction. As such, the origins of the freed slaves could not accurately be traced in most instances even to or via the Caribbean, let alone to specific areas of West Africa itself. "Return" would not be an appropriate description of the founding of the colonies of Sierra Leone and Liberia in West Africa in this sense. Further the state-making vision of the "returned" freed slaves was profoundly colonial.

The less expressed sentiment behind the vision that all freed slaves should live elsewhere than in the United States and United Kingdom is that the Blacks should be outside of the imperial territory unless they are enslaved: a manifestation of the nation as a white utopia. The freed slaves' presence "at home" in the settler colony is an untimely reminder of the key subvention capitalism required from the slaves themselves to get it going, which is free labor, just as it required "free" land from Indigenous peoples. The settler state, as a colonialist-capitalist Subject par excellence, does not admit to visible evidence of its dependence on exploitative labor practices with any grace.

Sierra Leone

After the American Revolutionary War, the British evacuated thousands of freed African-origin slaves and resettled them in Canadian and Caribbean colonies, and in London. In 1787, the Committee for the Freedom of the Black Poor founded a settlement in Sierra Leone in what was called the "Province of Freedom" or Granville Town, in a move that Emma Christopher terms, from the Committee's point of view, "a utopian antidote to slavery" (2008). About four hundred Blacks and sixty whites reached Sierra Leone on May 15, 1787. After they established Granville Town, most of the first group of colonists died from disease. As Isaac Land and Andrew Schocket put it, "their first attempt in 1787 was an economic and demographic failure" (2008). Note that the failure is attributed to the colonists, without any responsibility assigned to those seeking to move them "back" to West Africa, where they lacked appropriate resources, including local immunities. The sixty-four remaining colonists established a second Granville Town. The "resettlement" of freed slaves in Sierra Leone created essentially a group of neocolonists who, despite their shared "race" as Black, were not welcomed by the area's Indigenous inhabitants, although the Temne, Mende, and Sherbro peoples of the coast "were quite familiar with Europeans, having traded slaves and palm oil to them and been the subject of Christian missionary efforts for nearly two hundred years" (Land and Schocket 2008). The colonists did not view the Indigenous inhabitants as human, but as "uncivilized" others, following their own induction into colonialism, according to Christopher Fyfe (1962). Land and Schocket observe that:

> For all its revolutionary and utopian implications, the act of founding Freetown was an exercise of power, an exercise undertaken with very little consideration of the peoples already resident or living nearby. This uneasy dual legacy of freedom and colonialism presented political problems, not only for Sierra Leone's British rulers but also, and most acutely, for the emerging Krio population. By the last third of the nineteenth century, the Anglophilia and educational achievements of the Krio elite were increasingly mocked by racist Britons who sought to strip them of their offices and leadership positions, while their commercial acumen aroused envy and hostility on the part of other Africans who perceived them as rich interlopers. (2008)[9]

Further population of Sierra Leone followed, as well as the consequence of imperial dictates. Following the American Revolution, more than three thousand Black Loyalists (those loyal to the British Crown) had been settled in Nova Scotia, Canada, where they were finally granted land. They founded Birchtown, Nova Scotia, but harsh winters and racism made for a challenging existence. Thomas Peters, a freed slave originally from what is now Nigeria, together with British abolitionist John Clarkson, cofounded the Sierra Leone Company to relocate Black Loyalists who wanted to move to West Africa. In 1792, nearly twelve hundred persons from Nova Scotia crossed the Atlantic to build the settlement of Freetown. The settlers constructed Freetown in the architecture of the American South; they also undertook the sociopolitical building of the colony in the American culture with which they were familiar (Schama 2006). Throughout this settlement history, malaria, monsoon weather, and other challenges to their project decimated the settler populations. The British did not provide adequate basic supplies and building materials, and the settlers were threatened by reenslavement in the illegal slave trade. The Sierra Leone Company, controlled by London investors, refused to allow the settlers to take freehold of the land. The Crown subdued an ensuing revolt by bringing in forces of more than five hundred Maroons,[10] originally from Jamaica but also transported to Sierra Leone via Nova Scotia.

These Maroons had a complex history. When Britain took over Jamaica from Spain, the Spanish freed their slaves rather than have the British possess them. These freed slaves, together with run-away slaves, flourished in the highlands of Jamaica's interior. They were offered three pounds per recaptured slave by the British, income they used to buy luxury goods such as tea and sugar that they could not produce themselves: a preeminent example of the complexity of colonial capitalism, both in terms of exchange of money for slaves and commodities and slaves-as-commodities, and of the neocolonial aspect of structurally inducing the Maroons, themselves former slaves, to prey on current slaves, in a formation that, like the Americo-Liberians, colonization of what became Liberia, defies a simplistic Manichean allegory of colonizer versus colonized.

Indeed, the Maroons' nonidentification with the Jamaican slaves is the foundational characteristic of their identity, which means that, in their eyes, there was no ethical contradiction posed by their forming treaties with the British based on slave recovery numbers (Bilby 2005). When the Jamaican colonial authorities reduced the bounty for recaptured slaves from three to two pounds, hundreds of Maroons revolted in protest (Campbell 1988). In 1796, six hundred Maroons from Trelawney Town were transported to Halifax, Nova Scotia, as the British tried to export their Maroon adversaries. This was done without consultation of the current governor of Nova Scotia, Sir John Wentworth, and was based on the fact that Halifax was the nearest British port the British Navy transport ships would pass en route home (Fortin 2006) (Grant 2002).

The Maroons, unsurprisingly, were not enamored of either the weather or what they considered to be the menial labor of building or farming under British direction. The Crown employed their militaristic skills by sending them to Sierra Leone in 1800 to assist in pacifying the freed slaves of Freetown, the ones protesting against taxation. This constructs the perverse formulation of "troublesome" freed slaves, the Maroons, putting down another group of "troublesome" freed slaves in a postslavery global trajectory from Jamaica, to Canada, to Sierra Leone. These Maroons eventually became part of the community of resettled migrants to Sierra Leone. In later years, the Maroons regretted taking the governor's side in a conflict they did not at first understand. Even here, then, there is contradiction: "British authority against one group of Atlantic Africans could only be upheld through the misleading recruitment of other Atlantic Africans," comment Land and Schocket (2008).

On January 1, 1808, Thomas Ludlam, the governor of the Sierra Leone Company and a leading abolitionist, surrendered the company's charter. This ended its sixteen years of running the colony. However, British materialist interests were by no means absent. The British Crown reorganized the Sierra Leone Company as the African Institution, which was directed to improve the local economy. Its members represented both British who hoped to inspire local entrepreneurs and those with interest in the Macauley & Babington Company, which held the (British) monopoly on Sierra Leone trade (Lamont 1988; Diamond 1989).

Another perverse material "boost," as it were, to the inhabitants of the colony came in 1807, when, following the abolition of the slave trade, the Crown offered British Navy captains bounty for capturing and delivering now illegal slave trading ships to Freetown, where the slaves' value was assessed, the captain rewarded accordingly, and the slave ship captain and crew charged and tried. This, however, was an incentive both for slave traders to throw the slaves overboard when they knew they were being pursued and for British captains not to pursue a slaver who had thrown her cargo overboard, as the captain would not receive the reward for possession of the illegally taken slaves. It was more profitable for him to move on to attempt capture of a fully laden ship. Irrespective of the dire consequences of this move to contain illegal slavery, it resulted in thousands of formerly enslaved Africans being settled in Freetown. Having lost contact with their cultures of origin, these "receptives," as they were called, assimilated to the American project of social building in the colony, joining the erstwhile slaves from the American South and the Maroons (Sherwood 2007).

Liberia

Liberia has a history similarly affected by colonialist-capitalist management. In 1822, the American Colonization Society (ACS) began sending African American volunteers to the so-called Pepper Coast to establish a colony for freed African Americans. By 1867, the ACS had assisted in the movement of more than thirteen thousand Americans to Liberia (Burin 2005). These free African Americans came to identify themselves as Americo-Liberian, developing a social, political, and cultural tradition based on formative American political republicanism (Dunn-Marcos 2005;

Abaka 2007). The ACS was a private organization supported by prominent American politicians such as Abraham Lincoln, Henry Clay, and James Monroe. The ACS believed repatriation was preferable to the emancipation of slaves within American national territory (Abaka 2007; Sale 1997). This reflected the general belief that whites were superior to Blacks and that Blacks, therefore, could never live in equality alongside whites, and thus that their freedom in colonies over which they were to have political control would be better for them. It also offered the prospect of eliminating the "problem" of Blacks in (white) America, the constant reminder of the dependence of the colonialist-capitalist enterprise on mass slave labor forces. Similar organizations to the ACS established colonies named Mississippi in Africa and the Republic of Maryland, which were later annexed by Liberia. On July 26, 1847, the settlers issued a declaration of independence and promulgated a constitution based on the political principles of the U. S. Constitution, creating the independent Republic of Liberia (Adebajo 2002).

The leadership of the new nation consisted largely of the Americo-Liberians. The 1865 Ports of Entry Act prohibited foreign commerce with the inland tribes to encourage the growth of "civilized" values (Wegmann 2010), an explicit indication of the impropriety of settler–Indigenous communication. Indigenous Africans were understandably hostile to the colonists' incursions of their coast; in fact, Indigenous Africans were excluded from birthright citizenship in Liberia until as late as 1904. Wikipedia notes that, as the Republic of Liberia declared its independence on July 26, 1847, and was recognized by the United States as independent on February 5, 1862, "Liberia was the first African republic to proclaim its independence and is Africa's first and oldest modern republic. Along with Ethiopia, it was one of the two African countries to maintain its sovereignty during the Scramble for Africa" (n.d.). This statement erases the radical differences between the two states. Liberia's independence relied on its Americo-Liberian political identity and the neocolonial aspect of its development. Ethiopia was temporarily occupied only much later, during the Second World War, by Mussolini. Otherwise Ethiopia has been free of European colonization throughout its history, inspiring Rastafarianism in Jamaica in particular—yet another link to the history of the Maroons of Jamaica, many of whose descendants took up Rastafarianism avidly.

The comparison of Liberia and Ethiopia without referencing Ethiopia's long-standing independence is eerily reminiscent of the role Haiti plays in various racist iterations of the "Negro" and "African" problems. These are in actuality not separate problems, but related, white fantasies of the essential self-ungovernability of Blacks and of the resulting collapse of Black states. We can see this in the U.S. celebration of Liberia as the "true" inheritor of U.S. independence. Such independence has a white origin until it "goes wrong" due to the ungovernability, and lack of ability to govern, of Blacks. Robert Lansing, American secretary of state under Woodrow Wilson from 1915–1920, observes that:

> The experience of Liberia and Haiti shows that the African races are devoid of any capacity for political organization and lack genius for government. Unquestionably there is in them an inherent tendency to revert to savagery and to cast off the shackles of civilization which are irksome to their physical nature. . . . It is that which makes the negro problem practically unsolvable. (cited in Loveman 2010, 231)

This sentiment is echoed most recently by President Donald Trump in his reported reference to El Salvador, Haiti, and selected African states as "shithole" countries (Vitali, Hunt, and Thorp 2018).[11] The venom Haiti evinces in such rhetoric is a historically consistent response to its identity as the only state that successfully rebelled against slavery. Its punishment for doing so was to be cut off from international trade by the slave-owning states against which it rebelled and to be systematically impoverished for the "crime" of slave liberation.

Haiti

Unlike Sierra Leone and Liberia, the instantiation of Haiti as an independent state involves a rebellion against slavery. Not only did many slaves transit through Haiti, but also colonial French Haiti (then Saint Domingue) had more slaves than free Blacks or whites; the plantation economy depended on this labor. In the wake of the French Revolution in 1789, Haiti staged the only successful slavery rebellion worldwide starting in 1791, resulting in the establishment of the Republic of Haiti in 1804. However, in order to gain recognition from France and end crippling political and economic isolation, the new state was ordered to pay reparations for slave losses: the first time ever a military victory has been "rewarded" with a fine.

While the amount was decreased in 1838, the debt was not finally paid until 1947 (an act that foreshadowed the World Bank's use of structural adjustment to impoverish postcolonial economies in the seventies and eighties).

Haiti brings some crucial elements to the table in reading "African Ebola" now, despite the fact that these elements arise from repeatedly mutilated understandings of the facts. The first is the threat that Haiti posed and poses to Western modes of state governance, as an extant Black republic; the second is the difficulty of cultivating amnesia regarding slavery in the face of Haiti's existence; and the third is the place Haiti holds in the American imaginary as a place of both actual and cultural disease, represented respectively by poverty (inflicted by the U.S. and French empires), HIV/AIDS (this too has a colonially induced history), and the phenomenon of the zombie (which would not exist but for the slave trade). For now, let's address the racial threat Haiti poses to (white) American democracy.

From 1915 to 1934 the United States occupied Haiti to protect U.S. business interests on the island in line with Woodrow Wilson's Monroe Doctrine. In 1910/1911, the U.S. State Department had backed a consortium of American investors, assembled by the National City Bank of New York, in acquiring control of the Banquet National d'Haïti, the nation's only commercial bank and the government treasury. American President Woodrow Wilson sent 330 U.S. Marines to Port-au-Prince on July 28, 1915. The Haitian government had been receiving large loans from American and French banks over the past few decades and was growing increasingly incapable in fulfilling their "debt" repayment. Within six weeks of the occupation, the United States controlled Haitian customs houses and administrative institutions such as banks and the national treasury. The full measures by which the United States gained control of Haiti's governance are detailed by Paul Douglas (1927, 15–17). The excuse given for the invasion was the securing of the ports against supposed possible invasion by German submarines or French influence, a claim robustly dislodged by Douglas, who argues, contrary to Hans Schmidt (1995), that "there was virtually no danger of foreign intervention" (Douglas 1927, 21).

For the next nineteen years, advisers of the United States governed the country, enforced by the United States Marine Corps. The Marine Corps proved to be a predominantly racist and violent force, as was evidenced by their rampant drinking and sexual assault of local women. Further, the United States introduced compulsory work conscription to build Haiti's infrastructure, a much-hated resurrection of a form of slavery in its coercion of Indigenous inhabitants and their labor capacities. The National Association for the Advancement of Colored People (NAACP) secretary, Herbert J. Seligman, in the July 10, 1920, issue of *The Nation* magazine wrote:

> Military camps have been built throughout the island. The property of natives has been taken for military use. Haitians carrying a gun were for a time shot on sight. Machine guns have been turned on crowds of unarmed natives, and United States marines have, by accounts which several of them gave me in casual conversation, not troubled to investigate how many were killed or wounded.

In December 1929, according to Frank Senauth, "Marines in Les Cayes killed ten Haitian peasants during a march to protest local economic conditions. This led Herbert Hoover to appoint two commissions, including one headed by a former U.S. governor of the Philippines, William Cameron Forbes, which criticized the exclusion of Haitians from positions of authority in the government and constabulary, now known as the Garde d'Haïti" (2011, 31). By the time Hoover lost the election to Roosevelt in 1932, the American withdrawal from Haiti was in progress. In 1934 the United States left; however, Roosevelt had engineered the current Constitution of Haiti and the United States maintained control of Haiti's external finances until 1947.

Haiti's current economic crisis and political turmoil have their roots in the debt of one hundred and fifty million gold francs (later reduced to ninety million), which France imposed on the newborn republic with gunboats in 1825. The sum was supposed to compensate French planters for their losses of slaves and property during Haiti's 1791–1804 revolution, which gave birth to the world's first slavery-free, and hence truly free, republic. It is the only case in world history where the victor of a major war paid the loser reparations.

This extortion, perhaps more than any other nineteenth-century agreement, laid bare the hypocrisy of France's 1789 Declaration of the Rights of Man, modeled on the 1776 American Declaration of Independence, which proclaimed: "Men are born, and always continue, free and equal in respect of their rights" (National Assembly of France 1789). The United States, which assumed the debt in 1922, proved itself equally insincere in respecting this fundamental democratic principle for which it claims paternity. It took Haiti 122 years, until 1947, to pay off both the original ransom to

France and the tens of millions more in interest payments borrowed from French banks to meet the deadlines.

In 2003, Haiti became the world's first former colony to demand reparations (in the form of debt restitution) from a former colonial power. Then President Jean-Bertrand Aristide's government conservatively calculated the value of the restitution due at some $21.7 billion. Although the French parliament had unanimously approved a law recognizing the slave trade as a crime against humanity in 2001, just two years later France responded to Haiti's petition with fury. It angrily rejected the lawsuit and joined with Washington in brazenly fomenting a coup d'état against Aristide, who was ousted on February 29, 2004 (Joseph and Concannon 2015).

Aristide was removed from office after unrest starting in northern Haiti. Aristide and his bodyguard claimed that he was a victim of a new kind of coup d'état, a modern kidnapping by the United States. The United Nations Stabilization Mission was established in the wake of the coup d'état, consisting of Brazilian leadership, 2,366 military personnel, and 2,533 police, supported by international civilian personnel, a local civilian staff, and United Nations Volunteers, with the acronym MINUSTAH. In 2004, Tropical Storm Jeanne touched on the island, killing 3,006 people and leaving flooding and mudslides in its wake. In 2008, Tropical Storm Fay and Hurricanes Gustave, Hanna, and Ike left 331 dead and about eight hundred thousand in need of humanitarian aid. On January 12, 2010, at about 5 p.m., Haiti was struck by an earthquake registering 7.0 on the Richter scale. Thousands were killed and left homeless. To add insult to injury, cholera-infected waste was introduced via a MINUSTAH dump into the Artibonite, the country's main river. On October 4, 2016, Hurricane Matthew struck, leaving three thousand dead, further devastating the country's inadequate infrastructure, and ensuring growth in the cholera epidemic.[12]

The United Nations finally took some responsibility for the Nepalese strain of cholera being introduced to Haiti in 2011, admitting the Nepalese troops were "most likely" the source of the cholera, following epidemiological evidence of this fact (Cravioto et al. 2011). According to the CDC, over ninety-six hundred deaths and eight hundred thousand cases have been reported since 2010. Victims have made claims against the United Nations, to which it has responded, controversially, by proposing that remaining development dollars given since 2010 be used in development projects to support cholera victims; but cholera victims themselves want reparation, in an echo of the reparations for the slave reparation fines demanded by the Haitian government in 2013. In December 2016, General Secretary Ban Ki-Moon, while not admitting U.N. fault, apologized for the outbreak and spoke about the United Nations' "moral responsibility" for the Haitian epidemic (Sengupta 2016). The United Nations came up with a plan for $400 million to be raised voluntarily from member states, with $200 million going to survivors and $200 million going to communities directly affected by the epidemic. So far $9.22 million has been raised. In October 2017, MINUSTAH's mandate came to an end and was replaced by a much smaller force. MINUSTAH was plagued not only by the cholera outbreak but also by financial mismanagement, as well as rape by its Sri Lankan military contingent and other U.N. peacekeeping officials in a child sex ring and other forms of coerced sex against males and females.

Colonial Capitalism and the Biopolitical "Letting Die" of Postcolonial Illness as Debility

Haiti and the postcolonies of sub-Saharan Africa, including Sierra Leone and Liberia, share a history of colonial capitalism as a foundational sociopolitical determinant of health outcomes in those countries, a fact to which the cholera outbreak introduced by U.N. "assistance" after the 2010 earthquake testifies directly. Jasbir Puar has pointed out in her recent work on the Israeli–Palestinian conflict (2017) that, in this case, there is a biopolitics married not so much to slow death as to a state policy of maiming and stunting: since the Israelis cannot directly kill the Palestinians for political reasons, this kind of sustained attack on the biosocial infrastructure of Palestinians can be seen as the institutionalization of a biopolitics of debility. My argument would be that, in instituting debility, rather than death, as a biopolitical weapon, Israel is perhaps a spectacular instantiation of such a case, but *not* an exceptional one.

The institutionalization of a biopolitics of debility resurrects (if you will excuse the pun) not the spectral presence of a necropolitics or the politics of death, but one of life lived in constant proximity to radical socio*physical* vulnerability through the socio*political* (not social or socioeconomic, which are secondary) determinant of producing ongoing debility within an apparently disposable sector of the population. I say "apparently disposable" because colonialist-capitalist states, and indeed global capitalism itself, cannot exist without the labor of subjugated populations. This is not an instantiation, then, of Agamben's *bios* as opposed to *zoe*, the mere biological fact of life as opposed to the manner in which life is lived. In Agamben's work, *bios* (the biological fact of life) is characterized in his work, as Alexander Weheliye has pointed out (2014), by the racialized term of the *Musselman*, or *Muslim*.[13] This is the term that was used in the German concentration camps by inmates to refer to other inmates whose extreme thinness, frailty, and apathy marked them out as near death. Weheliye not only points out the racialized aspect of this term, but reminds us (2014, 85), citing the 1983 work of Zdzisław Ryn and Stanisław Kłodziński (in translation 2017), that the term *Musselman* did not necessarily mean those for whom the next episode was the gas chamber. At any time, 50–80 percent of concentration camp prisoners could be referred to as *Musselman*. That is to say, prisoners did not reach the state of *Musselman* once on their way to death, but "moved in and out of being-*Musselman*." They became exceptionally frail, recovered, and then reentered a critical stage of frailty repeatedly.

Weheliye's analysis is constructive in that it demonstrates the desire of onlookers of illness to wish away the sufferer in a move that dislocated debility into death. It would be easier, the logic goes, for us to think of Holocaust survivors as entering an extreme state of frailty only once, rather than as suffering repeated attacks and barely recovering from them, but nevertheless not dying. What Weheliye makes visible is not the horror of murder alone, but the horror of ongoing debility. Debility has been and continues to be a condition of life for many in the postcolonies, not an exceptional state. Hence it does not conform to the binary of that life that is associated with culture (in Agamben's terms, the way in which life is lived, *zoe*, and that which is lived at the level of bare life, *bios*). Mbembe describes the letting die of "disposable" populations in the postcolony as a process of making the political subject (as opposed to object) live, in a structure that precisely links the Foucauldian sovereign powers to make live and to let die (2003, 27). Political "objects," disposable populations, die in order precisely to make sovereign political subjects live. The death of the other is not incidental to the instantiation of the sovereign subject; the thriving of the sovereign—or in my terms, colonialist-capitalist—subject actually depends upon the death of that other. In Mbembe's formulation, the object of the exercise of sovereignty is not aimed at autonomy, but the exercise or the performance of power: "To exercise sovereignty is to exercise control over mortality and to define life as the deployment and manifestation of power" (13), and "the generalized instrumentalization of human existence and the material destruction of human bodies and populations" is the central project of power (14).

The context of this is in Mbembe's work is explicitly the postcolony, and he pays due attention, following Foucault, to the preeminence of race in the determination of disposability. However, reading the postcolony as an extended domain of Agamben's "state of exception," as Mbembe does, may overlook Henry Giroux's point: What is at stake is a sense of disposability, rationalized in terms of the economy rather than those of sovereign power, applicable in scenes such as Hurricane Katrina (2006, 7–8). The focus on *necropolitics* (Mbembe's term for the politics of death) should not steer us away from the politics of slow death, which is not captured by Agamben's *zoe* versus *bios*. The politics of debility means living in states of instrumentalization that exceed Agamben's "state of exception" (instrumentalization is not an exception) and create situations in which neither *zoe* nor *bios* applies as a category. The debilitated are neither *Musselmanner*, the almost dead, or thriving; the debilitated include those with chronic conditions, with ongoing vulnerability to further erosion of physical security and death looming, rather than necessarily imminent.

We see necropolitics of a sort at work in the fact that the mass of Black Ebola victims of the 2014 epidemic instantiate the individual subject of the non-Black Ebola survivor, such as Nina Pham or Kent Brantly, enabling his or her naming. Yet once again, letting die to make live is only one end of the spectrum: maiming, or introducing debility in the postcolonial subject, is conceivably a far more politically sustainable way to make the settler capitalist thrive. In view of this, I propose using Puar's concept to rewrite Mbembe's formulation as follows: the disabling of the disposable "other" is not incidental to the colonialist-capitalist; the quality of life of the latter actually depends on the debility, but not the genocide, of the disposable; although the risk of death is inherent in, and calculated as acceptable loss for, the working of a politics of debility. This means the politics of debility depends on a (non)ethic of infinite substitutability, because the debilitated population is not as a whole disposable, in that it is required for colonial capitalism to thrive; but those who constitute it do not need to be consistent, merely substitutable.

The Practice of "Rescue" Medicine in the Global South

In spite of the fact that Anderson wrote "Where Is the Postcolonial History of Medicine?" over two decades ago (1998), it would seem we are still "writing a minor literature," which has deeply problematic, actual effects, as Western medicine is assumed to be both normalized and superior to Indigenous traditions and cultures of healing and wellness on all counts, as Alan Bleakley, Julie Brice Browne, and John Bligh point out:

> Western medicine and medical techniques are being exported to all corners of the world at an increasing rate. In a parallel wave of globalization, Western medical education is also making inroads into medical schools, hospitals and clinics across the world. Despite this rapidly expanding field of activity, there is no body of literature discussing the relationship between postcolonial theory and medical education.
>
> We need to develop greater understanding of the relations between postcolonial studies and medical education if we are to prevent a new wave of imperialism through the unreflecting dissemination of conceptual frameworks and practices which assume that "metropolitan West is best." (2008, 266)

Add to this, first, the current focus in medical education on "cultural competence" as a means of communicating effectively with communities from cultures other than the Western scientific and, second, the current rage for global health experience among medical students. Firstly, "cultural competence" has nothing to do with cultural competence in the sense that it constitutes an instrumentalist set of tools for more efficiently conveying the authority and superiority of Western medicine in contexts in which such superiority could be questioned by Indigenous and postcolonial communities. The CDC takes its definition of cultural competency from the U.S. Department of Health and Human Services, Office of Minority Health, which assumes that the patient is defined above all as a "consumer" of Western health services, despite the document's apparent concern with identifying the health provider's own beliefs as a potential barrier to positive outcomes in situations where the aforementioned "consumer" is of a minority.[14] Following Anderson, cultural competence pedagogies do not ask, "what is colonial about Western medicine in any setting?," and they assume that the Western-trained healer is able to develop competence in the culture of the other, or at least, able to develop sufficient "skill" to impose Western medicine authoritatively in the cultural setting of the other under the sign of "cultural competence."

As I have noted elsewhere, the practice of medicine in conjunction with the allures of the postcolonial exotic creates a fatal medical neo-imperialism. I spent three years of my childhood in Lesotho, an independent nation enclosed by South Africa, in a mission hospital where my father was the only doctor for forty thousand square miles, and we lived in the geographical center of the country along the infamously dangerous "Mountain Road." We would get well-meaning donations to the hospital that made us laugh and cry at the same time: an unbelievably expensive piece of a heart transplant machine, which we then had to find a buyer for to garner the income for the hospital's needs, and hundreds of disposable needles that had already been used. The postage expended to get them to us we could well have deployed for real needs. Who, one wonders, thinks that one can reuse disposable needles? And what population "deserves" such "care"?

Lesotho depends on charity, migrant labor, and garment work, as well as subsistence farming. The country is among the group of "Low Human Development" countries (ranked 168 of 191 on the Human Development Index as classified in the United Nations *Human Development Insights* in 2023). The current 2023 life-expectancy figure is 55.65 years, and while adult literacy rose as high as 81.02 percent in 2021, the infant mortality that year was still high, with 55.183 deaths per thousand babies (Macrotrends 2023). According to 2021 estimates, the prevalence of HIV was about 20.9 percent, one of the highest in the world, with 290,000 living with HIV, 74,000 new HIV infections, 4,500 deaths, and 81 percent of infected adults on highly active antiretroviral drugs (HAART) (UNAIDS 2021).

I once had a discussion with a colleague who was taking groups of students over to a Canadian-sponsored HIV clinic in Botswana; he figured he could keep the clinic going through rotations of medical students and locums from Canada indefinitely. He was mirroring the approach of Philip Berger, who worked under the auspices of OH Africa (an NGO associated with the Ontario Hospital Foundation) at the Basotho clinic he had set up in late 2004. The clinic was due for a normal transfer from foreign to Basotho government control, as was recognized by the Canadians themselves. However, as the takeover loomed, Berger and OH Africa warned of a "life or death" crisis at the clinic, due to the withdrawal of the Canadian staff, a refusal of the Basotho national government to pay for fifteen local workers, and fear that integration of the clinic into the hospital would lead to stigma-related avoidance and a diminishment in care standards.

The clinic at one point boasted of having attracted fifty Canadians to its locale. This raises the questions of what programs were in place for the transfer of skills from the Canadians to the local medical staff and what plans were made by the clinic for its eventual transfer to the central government, a condition by which the clinic had operated with the Basotho government's permission. HAART administration becomes a complicated business only when rarer forms of resistance to regimes appear. However, this is used as a form of threat in an instantiation of Canadian superiority in the language of the letter written to the Basotho government by the OH Africa and Dr. Berger:

> Now, after a dispute with the Lesotho government, the Canadian donors are warning of a nightmare scenario. Patients could die, they say, and the clinic could spark a public-health crisis by spreading drug-resistant HIV strains across the border to South Africa.
>
> Health professionals at the clinic are already beginning to leave, and key programs are disintegrating. "This is a life-and-death urgent matter for the people of the region, said Philip Berger, a Toronto doctor who specializes in AIDS treatment and has worked at the Lesotho clinic as recently as December. (York 2010)

This implies that new strains of resilience are not spreading within South Africa itself and do not often come *from* there, a patently empty claim: indeed, I'd be more worried about such strains coming into Lesotho, not going from there into South Africa, as South Africa has a far more advanced HIV/AIDS system for detecting and dealing with such strains, and a far larger population in which to develop them. Further, we have considerable experience now of how to destigmatize HIV clinics within a hospital setting, such as making sure they are integrated with pre- and post-natal care, and are not "stand alone," so that patients visiting them cannot be identified as HIV-positive or not.

My main point, not a new one, but not a persuasive one, apparently, is that intercultural skills transfer to local professionals should be part and parcel of the plan. I understand that there would be resistance on the part of clinic-goers to the change in care, which may be less personalized, require further travel (a huge problem in the service of the highlands in Lesotho in particular), seem less "high tech," and therefore be perceived to be less effective. Working within a hospital administration poses barriers not encountered in individual, specialized clinics—no question—as I experienced in my own attempts to integrate NGO rape-crisis clinics into hospitals in rural KZN. But what does it mean to develop clinics in Lesotho and Botswana that effectively depend on rotating medical staff trained in Canada to do locum and fixed-term work at the clinics? As the minister of health of Lesotho, Mphu Ramatlapeng, put it in an e-mail to *The Globe and Mail*: "They experienced a very high turnover of staff and they failed to meet certain targets.... They failed to integrate the clinic services with the services of the main hospital. They also failed to assist us with decentralized services to the clinics" (cited in York 2010).

The most important services communities need when members are on antiretroviral (ARV) treatments are the complex but nontechnical skills to: persuade a mother not to give her drugs to her husband or another family member because they won't go for testing; ensure that the family (however constituted) has access to the right kinds of foods and good quality water to sustain taking ARVs (both food and water are a problem in Lesotho); explain the importance of condom usage to discordant couples and those at risk of cross-infection of different strains; prevent mother-to-child transmission; negotiate traditional healer integration with ARV regimes, and appraise patients of the possibility of resistance and its symptoms and postresistance options. These are all public health and interpersonal skills services best offered in Sesotho in the context of its extremely high poverty and unemployment rates, and with an understanding of the modern history of the country as, until recently, a men's (and now, increasingly) women's labor camp for South African industry.

Canadians and other Westerners founding clinics in the global South are often not attentive to the repetition of the hubris of colonialism and the cost of that hubris to local populations. At issue is the lack of the sustainability of foreign interventions, just as it was when the Belgians failed to train successors when they pulled out of the Congo on June 30, 1960. The ensuing development of the postcolonial state, in part by expatriate Haitians, is the factor to which Peter Piot and others, such as Oliver Pybus, infectious disease specialist and evolutionary biologist at the University of Oxford, attribute the introduction of HIV to Haiti. Returning expatriates brought the genetic forerunner of the current epidemic back to Haiti with them from the DRC (Faria et al. 2014). As Pybus, Andrew J. Tatem, and Phillipe Lemey point out, "the effects of global mobility upon the genetic diversity and molecular evolution of pathogens are under-appreciated and only beginning to be understood" (2015). Also at stake are postnatal care units and other physical areas of the hospital that offer highly unstigmatized and long-standing services, including Tuberculosis services, which have a long history in Lesotho owing to the migrant mineworkers. HIV drug resistance (HIVDR) is an increasing threat to treatment globally. The development of laboratory capacities for testing goes hand-in-hand with country ownership and governance mechanisms to ensure sustainable responses to HIVDR (WHO 2017a; note objective 4). Further, there are community resources that go unrecognized in the enshrining of Western medicine as the gold standard. Before the availability of ARVs in South Africa, Sangoma (traditional healer) Benghu reminded me once, the folks at King Edward VIII Hospital in Durban used to tell HIV-positive patients from the Valley of a Thousand Hills to "go home to die." It was the traditional healers who supported them in their quest as to *how to live* with the disease. Conceiving the ill postcolonial citizen as purely a victim is rife with fantasies of humanitarianism, technological superiority, and the zeal of Western medicine to practice under the sign of the exotic tropic.

What might a way out of this conundrum be?

The Zombie as Revenant

The absent figure in the Halloween costume is that of the unspeakable Ebola victim. Thus, while biohazard containment costumes abounded in popularity in October 2014, their twin costume, so to speak, was (thankfully) absent, as noted above. The Ebola victim, despite the potential of the stereotype of Ebola as a (misnamed) hemorrhagic fever to offer Halloween costumes of gruesome creativity matched only by inexorable bad taste, was present by her/his spectacular, racialized absence. If there were instances of Halloween makeup verging on the popular notion of Ebola as a spectacular hemorrhagic fever inaccurately perpetuated by texts such as Richard Preston's 1994 *The Hot Zone,* these occupy a pleasurable distance from the actual fact of the person who dies from Ebola.[15] Makeup itself suggests containment through its manipulation of a stable face, a stable body in costume, rather than the unpredictably effluent body of the dying person, in which the actual moment of death is buried in days and hours of deep suffering. If this absent figure has an actual correlative, it would perhaps be Thomas Eric Duncan, a Black American with a reportedly thick West African accent who became infected on a visit to West Africa and later died in a Dallas hospital, having been neither treated with the drug cocktail offered to white survivors nor transfused with the blood of a survivor, both interventions demonstrated to improve the victim's chances of survival (Karimi and Shoichet 2014). Ironically, despite the panic in the Unites States over Ebola, the failure to recognize the disease "on home turf" and the related failure of provision of services killed Duncan.

It is with the absent figure of the Ebola zombie that I wish to conclude. The zombie becomes tied in with the Ebola victim in the strange reports of Ebola victims who come back to life after they are dead, notably two women from the Nimba Country of Liberia. While this is obviously "fake news," so to speak (they were likely falsely pronounced dead in the height of the epidemic), what is notable is the facility with which citizens latched onto Ebola hysteria in the United Kingdom and the United States. I argued above that the Ebola-containment Halloween costume and its absent other, the racialized Ebola victim, speaks a certain history, that of a colonialist-capitalist regime in which biomedicine prevents whites being harmed (and, one might argue, from "susceptibiltiy" to nonheteronormative gender formations, considering the gendered nature of the outfits), while consigning actual victims in need of help to the speculative region of an invisible, unspeakable, fantastically dystopian, and disease-riddled, and indeed a disposable, "Africa."

In the engaging, telling, and often meticulous genre of zombie studies, the zombie is traced through its Haitian original in voodoo, through its appearances in the rampant genre of the zombie movie via George Romero, through to its appearance not as the living dead, but those who live *as if* they were dead: those who stave off a sense of limited subjectivity, for example, through rampant consumerism. Here the zombie is not the Ebola victim per se, but its supposedly privileged other, the consumer who buys the Halloween costume in a putative but genuine attempt to stave off threats to an absolute sovereignty. This desire has its adult expression in the survivalists who bought real Ebola/hazmat-containment suits to the tune of thousands of dollars, despite the fact that their potential exposure to Ebola was nil.[16]

This phenomenon speaks to the mixture of desire and fear we see in such costuming against a future threat that comes from a racialized elsewhere. The telling aspect of this scene lies, as rehearsed previously, in the fear of diminished white sovereignty, of diminished consumer colonialism, of the failure of rationality in the history of the West, and of the retreat of colonial capitalism in the face of a history of the Black/slave/debilitated/sick subject as revenant. The figure of the zombie comes to us as revenant in the spectral politics of Ebola through the sufferers "raised from the dead" and through the smiling faces of apparently perfectly healthy subjects wearing Ebola makeup, as in the Dutch campaign for Doctors without Borders that sought to raise awareness of the disease through celebrity "Ebola selfies."

Bringing an effluent eye to the persistent figure of the zombie enables us to see a weakness in Roberto Esposito's immunological biopolitics. Esposito views modernity and biopolitics through the lens of immunity, which he opposes to community. In modernity, he argues, the need to defend against others rather than build community expansively reigns: As Nietzsche saw clearly, he argues, "what we call 'modernity' is nothing but the meta-language that allowed [us] to respond in immunitarian terms to several demands of preventive protection, . . . when the promises of transcendent salvation were failing" (2013, 97). That is to say, when secularism threatens the afterlife as it is conceived in Judeo-Christian terms, technology offers the promise of survivability in this life through immunization, not simply as medical practice, but as a foundational paradigm for sovereign human life in a secular field. If in premodern times the sovereign never dies—only the king, who occupied the position of the sovereign, dies—in secular modernity, the Human can be resurrected as actual sovereign, not just as occupying the position of the sovereign, through the paradigm of immunization.

As the paradigm of immunization helps us to grasp the structural link between modernity and biopolitics, the paradigm of autoimmunization lets us establish the relation, as well as the element of discontinuity, between modern biopolitics and Nazi thanatopolitics, where thanatopolitics is "a politics of death . . . stand[ing] in opposition to biopolitics and its affirmative instantiations of life itself":

Regarding [thanatopolitics], . . . not only the racial politics of the German people became the principle aim of German politics—in a way that affected their survival to the death of its external and internal enemies—but at some point, when defeat seemed inevitable, the order of its self-destruction was given. In this case the immunitarian system assumed a fully auto-immunitarian connotation and biopolitics came to perfectly coincide with thanatopolitics. (Esposito 2013, 87)

As Esposito also characterized thanatopolitics, it is "operationalized as the progression of life through increasing the 'circle of death'" (2008, 110).

However, first let us remind Esposito that the modernity of which he speaks is inflected with colonialism, without which Esposito's modernity is unthinkable (as is Foucault's, although Foucault is far more aware of the fact). Then let us return to the fact that the refusal of the opposition between *zoe* and *bios* under the sign of contemporary global capitalism is negotiated by the mobilization not of mass death to enable biopolitical life, but mass debility: the debilitation of the other is not incidental to the colonialist-capitalist. The quality of life of the latter actually depends on the debility of the former, as I rephrased Puar earlier. The zombie as the one who consumes without awareness of its state of unawareness in this scenario would reflect the disability of colonialist-capitalist citizens. What can we "let be born" if we conceive as *reflexive* rather than *undirectional* the connection between the Subject who lets the "object" live debilitated and the objectsubject who lives debilitated? And what if the form that reflexivity takes is that of the zombie? Rather than a binary opposition between racialized utopias supported by capitalist biomedical regimes and their dystopian others, the literally disarticulated biopolitical regime of systemic debility in the postcolony, we could attend instead to the zombie as a figure that itself *disarticulates the binary between the citizen and the debilitated,* defined as available for disablement and death. The disarticulation of the citizen–zombie binary and the disposable has the potential to lead us to some preliminary understanding of Esposito's politics of immunity as potentially reciprocal, and therefore not a politics of immunity at all, but one of a materially presented discursive possibility of eluding the immunity–community binary, in Esposito's terms: a fragile opening onto a positively co-constituted community of effluence comprising the citizen-subject and the effluent-subject, the latter of which is not defined by an availability for further debility, but embodied self-knowledge of how to read both the separation and the interaction of biological disease vectors and sociopolitical vectors. To put it bluntly: how does one take the observation of the isiZulu lady I interviewed in KZN seriously? How does one listen to her with an effluent ear?

The kind of sovereign Foucault appeals to is a historical reality but a current fiction: very few sovereigns are left who singularly have the power to make die and let live in an uncomplicated gesture of power, as Mbembe points out. More relevant, however, is the material presence of utopian nationalisms playing themselves out over history in the face of the hypersovereignty of multinational capital. In this respect, the inheritors of the white utopian dream of colonialist-capitalist triumphalism—some of whom are not white, of course—are indeed haunted by the specter of the slave. For, in making the human a commodity, the irrevocable decision to commit to the law of commodification, rather than the value of extramaterial meanings, was made, and the human-who-does-not-produce (or oversee production) was rendered available for debility; as David Harvey argues, "sickness is defined broadly under capitalism as inability to work" (2000, 106).

The refusal to respond to the call of Haiti for reparations for slavery thus speaks both to the hypocrisy of the nation-state (France and the United States, in this case), with its commitment to humans as commodities (not making amends for slavery) even as it claims publicly to be against the idea, and to the nation-state's own diminishment of its supposedly sovereign subjectivity in the face of the disarticulation of colony and capital, as global economic power moves away from its traditional western European and North American shores and financial exchange migrates out of the power of the state under the sign of capitalism. This disarticulation of nation-state and capital can be seen as systemic debility only from the perspective of the colonialist-capitalist zombie, filled with the fantasy of a good life with no repercussions or debts, financial or ethical: a perfect, walled, politics of immunity. But, for those living in actual conditions of colonialist-capitalist-induced debility, not all of them in the traditionally recognized settler colonies, the diminishment of colonialist-capitalist sovereignty is not necessarily a marker of a new vulnerability. It offers an opportunity, perhaps, for a more equitable sharing of vulnerability across nations and races, a more equitable cohabitation in conditions of effluent community; but this outcome is uncertain and deeply fragile, analogous to but not the same as the fragility of the *Musselman* in its ebb and flow.

In any event, one difference between the agency of Ebola and the agency of the biopolitical human remains: Ebola may often kill its victims in places of colonial capitalism, through underdeveloped medical systems and supports; but it is not the kind of subject that does so in acts of racialized, biopolitical violence that depend on the sustaining of debility, the kinds of acts with which my interviewee is so familiar and of which she has an embodied knowledge. As long as the postcolony remains host to colonialist-capitalist legacies of human agency, a productive infrastructure of postcolonial debility serves the racialized ends of neocolonialist, "utopian"/immunitarian politics. Indeed, factors in being infected by Ebola and dying from it are colonialist-capitalist in nature, having to do with the structural violence of the underdevelopment of health infrastructures in West Africa. Yet, as I demonstrate in the next chapter, subjects in excess of the state are not bound to the immunitarian injunction to create community only through exclusion, and thus can enable persistence against the politics of immunity that Esposito so claustrophobically describes, in which what is feared must be immunized against, pitting the Subject against the other and framing subjectivity as, tellingly, impossibly against community, to the extent that the threatened community offs itself before it is defeated, as in the example of Germany given by Esposito.

In the following chapter, I discuss two novels from the perspective of an effluence-inspired critical ear, as a kind of listening to the isiZulu *gogo* (older lady), my Underberg-based interlocutor. Jennifer Haigh's novel *Heat and Light* is expert at describing Esposito's immunitarian politics in fictional terms, while Masande Ntshanga's *The Reactive* describes an effluent alternative. In *The Reactive*, Lindanathi, the narrator, assigns a deep value to the *inability* to help the other in certain situations on the grounds of, first, a lack of knowledge of the situation, where such lack of knowledge is not registered as fear and, second, the notion that the desire to help the other is more often than not a fleeing from attention to the inadequacies of the self. While this plays out on an interpersonal level in relation to the characters in Lindanathi's narrative, it is also structurally connected to the dangers of humanitarian investments within the violence of a system in which medicine is privatized, and therefore offered in enormous acts of "generosity" rather than provided as a common good. The transactional quality of both financial and humanitarian exchange, we discover, are part of an economy to which effluent communities can show signs of persistence, not in a mass utopian vision that comes under the sign of Resistance with a capital "R," but in fragile, patchy, but consistent production of evidence of how one might envision living outside colonialist-capitalist value. This practice has intermittent success, where success is defined as the ability to live on the margins in a state of persistence against colonialist-capitalist structural violence, not in the white-zombie terms of the ability to accrue material value from the margins.

3

Addiction and Its Formations under Capitalism

Refusing the Bubble and Effluent Persistence

This chapter addresses the connections between colonial capitalism and substance abuse in a comparative reading of a novel from Pennsylvania, Jennifer Haigh's 2016 *Heat and Light,* and one from South Africa, Masande Ntshanga's *The Reactive,* from the same year. The comparison highlights both the ubiquity but also the uneven development of global capitalism and the differential effects of this uneven development on the speakability of the failures of capitalism within distinct cultures. While Haigh uses the mousetrap game, described in the next section, as an implicit reflection of the entrapment of workers in capitalism, Ntshanga's protagonist, Lindanathi, escapes capitalism's constraints by refusing to play according to its relentless rules. He decides on a different set of values, as we shall see. At the same time, comparison raises the question of whether the possibility of opting out of capitalism, to the extent possible, is more or less an available opportunity, depending upon capitalism's saturation of any given local community's *habitus,* or ways of being in the world. *Habitus* is Pierre Bourdieu's word, described by L. Wacquant as "the way society becomes deposited in persons in the form of lasting dispositions, or trained capacities and structured propensities to think, feel and act in determinant ways, which then guide them" (2005, 316). The comparison I make in this chapter has implications for thinking about substance use and capitalism as sharing an all-consuming culture. Indeed, whether substance is used or abused opens the question of whether capitalism is itself useful or abusive.

What Is the Mousetrap?

In 2016, Jennifer Haigh published the novel *Heat and Light,* which concerns the dependence on extractive industries for energy, specifically in Pennsylvania. One of the characters, Wesley Peacock, belongs to a family that does not evacuate the Three Mile Island area when he is a child; he later dies of cancer, which cannot be linked with certainty to the infamous radiation leak,[1] but which he is convinced is the cause of his cancer. He is not evacuated because he is neither in the womb nor a preschooler. He is home-schooled. He does not want to go to school; he is addicted to the care of his mother and envisions as desirable the position of the boy in the 1976 movie *Boy in the Plastic Bubble* (directed by Randall Kleiser and starring John Travolta, Glynnis O'Connor, and Robert Reed). He remembers the boy actor explaining that he "is not so unhappy in here as all of you think" (Haigh 2016, 148). I propose that this bubble represents the bubble of Western medical care and its associated *cordon sanitaire* as I described it in terms of health care as a colonial-settler white's right. The bubble, then, is metonymically connected to systems of colonial capitalism within which a predominantly privately funded health-care system sits (as opposed to the full public system of, say, Canada, or the dual public-private system of the United Kingdom). In an otherwise realist novel, Wesley Peacock comes back from the dead to continue to assert that his death has been the result of the Three Mile Island leak. This suggests that the bubble-(white)-citizen relation is one of contract: if those who believe in, and thereby make, the bubble support it, they expect protection from it. In short, Wesley Peacock feels betrayed: he took little risk—he even refuses having children, wanting himself to continue to be the apple of his spouse's eye—and therefore expected no negative consequences to result from his choices. In a microcosm of this context, as a child he plays a game in which a series of dice throws between players lead to the construction of a trap, the end of the game being the release of a cage from the top of a post to trap an "unsuspecting mouse" (149). This indicates that he, like other characters in the novel, does not see that, when the bubble of colonial-settler capitalism bursts, the fallout will land on him. This happens to other characters in the novel, some of whom recognize that the bubble is broken and some who see their misfortune as simply unlucky. That is to say, the bubble breaks whether those party to its contract recognize it or not.

At the time of the Three Mile Island leak, Wesley's mother keeps the windows shut because the hydrogen bubble, that other actuality, is growing, as if windows are adequate protection against radiation. Ironically, enough, the neighbor asks Wesley's mother if she has lead windows, as these are said to help keep radiation out. Although the text doesn't relate whether the Peacocks do or do not have lead windows, or whether the glass or the paint may be lead, current EPA regulations consider the dispersal of lead dust to be so harmful, especially to children, that a lead-safe qualification for lead-detected windows is required for their removal (Environmental Protection Agency 2017). Once again, what is assumed by the characters to save them, whether the bubble or lead windows, is actually, in the event, detrimental to them. Indeed, environmental security is unobtainable and emotional security radically scarce in *Heat and Light*: whatever one does to protect oneself from being entrapped in the metonymical bubble engages one further in a network of circumstances one cannot overcome through that much-vaunted power of the individual in the American dream. Hence the microcosm of the mousetrap. Like all dice games, the game of the novel has some characters on the upswing and others on the downswing, but all of their actions are determined by, or damagingly contained by, the dictates of colonial capitalism. The trap does not need to be released on the unsuspecting mouse; it's just that the unsuspecting mouse may suddenly realize it is in the trap.

In this chapter I juxtapose two globally different sites of colonial capitalism: Pennsylvania for Haigh's *Heat and Light* and Cape Town for Ntshanga's *The Reactive*. The methodology for such a comparison could broadly be identified as an exploration of the theory postulated by the Warwick Research Collective (WReC) in their 2015 *Combined and Uneven Development*, that world literature manifests, in generic terms, Trotsky's theory of combined but uneven development. In this theory, as I noted in my introduction, the world is globally under capitalist sway, but the movement toward this capitalist "state" is highly differentially, or more precisely, unevenly manifest. The WReC's critique does not assume a hierarchy in which the most developed state is the most efficient or morally superior, or even the desired goal. In this sense, the core of *Combined and Uneven Development* is not implicated in the notion that the goal of development is an unambiguously good thing: the WReC is explicit in its disavowal evaluations of development that remain untouched by colonialist-capitalist critique.

Thus the kind of literary "Great Tradition" proposed by F. R. Leavis can be seen, in WreC's terms, as a manifestation of the Western European genre of the novel intersecting with particular stages of colonialist-capitalist development (Leavis 1948). The same would go for Ian Watt's 1957 history of the novel: the consolidation of the individual as character, protagonist, or solid citizen we see in Daniel Defoe and Samuel Richardson is consonant with the individual as commanding human-rights we see in Joseph Slaughter's 2007 bildungsroman. These are very broad strokes, however. Here I wish to draw specifically on the kind of airlessness or hopelessness of the subjects in Haigh's bubble—all of whom are affluent, materially speaking, when compared with their effluent counterparts in *The Reactive*—to demonstrate how genres and communities of effluence, despite their "ungrievability" in Judith Butler's terms (2009), demonstrate options for different formations of the subject, and thus different futures for the subject, that are foreclosed in the world of Haigh's meticulous bubble, which ruthlessly demonstrates the need for alternative formations of the subject.

The Myth of the Subject—On Judith Butler's Precarity

In Butler's formation of precarity, she claims: "Precarity designates that politically induced condition in which certain populations suffer from failing social and economic networks of support and become differentially exposed to injury, violence, and death" (2009, 25). That state has, however, taught us that "to be protected from violence by the nation-state is to be exposed to the violence wielded by the nation-state.... Precarity... characterizes that politically induced condition of maximized precariousness for populations exposed to arbitrary state violence who often have no option but to appeal to that state from which they require protection" (26). In other words, "To rely on the nation-state for protection from violence is precisely to exchange one potential violence for another. There may, indeed, be few other choices," Butler claims (26). Further, Butler understands that the human-rights framework cannot render life *not precarious*, since the only form of life the human-rights regime recognizes is one that (already) has a status of a person: one who has the actual potential to be, or is involved in, the *business* of creating the good life, both symptom and diagnosis of which can be only that material reality that we recognize as possession. She also argues, and I agree, that the conditions of life are deeply interdependent. She intends this in the sense of human interdependency, whereas I would include nonhuman animals and natural and built environments, with all their entanglements, alongside the human.

Colonial capitalism renders the interdependency that is the precondition of sustaining life invisible in the sleight of hand in which to choose to thrive is to make the choices about what kinds of products are most likely to get one further up the corporate ladder of the business of the good life. That is to say, colonial capitalism, represented by the bubble, likes to make itself invisible, just as the bubble in the film is glass. One practices reliance on the bubble while *not* noticing it's there. I suggest a related elision exists in Butler's work, an elision that speaks to the U.S. context in which she primarily works: the confusion of the state with colonial capitalism. That is to say, one can replace the bubble, as I have described it, with the state in her observations about the state. For example, in *Heat and Light*, to be protected by the violence of the bubble (its exclusions) is to become subject to the violence of the bubble, when the apparent protection it provided turns out to betray the protected. In literal terms, one can also turn Butler's thinking on its head in relation not only to the vulnerable but also to the supposedly protected or proper citizen. The supposed beneficiaries of the state are provided security and assume, once a Black Lives Matter moves in, that they are suddenly unprotected. That is to say, one is made all the more *less* free if one's security is both granted and threatened by the state, in a situation in which the state is in fact complicit in fusing together the rights of the citizen and the rights of the consumer, literally *con*fusing them. This stands both for the improper citizen, the ungrievable, and the proper citizen, like Wesley Peacock. In this context, we need to go a step beyond Butler's comments on the state in *Frames of War*:

> Without grievability, there is no life, or, rather, there is something living that is other than life. Instead, "there is a life that will never have been lived," sustained by no regard, no testimony, and ungrieved when lost. The apprehension of grievability precedes and makes possible the apprehension of precarious life. Grievability precedes and makes possible the apprehension of the living being as living, exposed to non-life from the start. (2009, 15)

Communities of the effluent live outside or on the margins of the state in its assumption of the good life as everyone's business. Many postcolonial communities, Indigenous, and those otherwise rendered marginal are persistent precisely because they *no longer or never did believe in the authority and/or capacity of the state to provide basic security, let alone any good life*. Furthermore, such communities do not mistake, or confuse, the state with colonial capitalism, although they find ways of speaking the relations between the two, as we shall see. Butler's theory depends on an optics of recognition that overlooks the affirmation of community, and the grievability and other forms of solidarity that accompany intercommunity bonds within effluent communities. That is to say, Butler remarks on the human who commands rights within the bubble as able to grieve other humans who command rights within the bubble, but as unable to grieve precarious life, which would include communities of effluence outside the purview of the bubble, those who are outside first because the phenomenal cost of a medical intervention such as the bubble would not be borne by the state or capitalism on their behalf, and second because they don't believe in the bubble and have never contributed to its myth. In this respect, Butler describes Kelly Oliver's (2001) understanding of the weaknesses of *recognition as opposed to affirmation,* where recognition relies on the dominant culture (think inside the bubble) to recognize the ungrievable in a gesture of liberal, paternalistic inclusion (think outside the bubble). However, Butler's paradigm completely overlooks intereffluent affirmation, or affirmation between subjects excluded from the bubble, or subjects who have excluded themselves from the bubble.

Oliver critiques the politics of recognition in its limitations as a liberal form of inclusion: one can be borne witness to only if the subject who commands human rights *already* acknowledges the other's right to recognition. Thus Oliver argues that the other—say, in my terms, the effluent community as subject, the outside-the-bubble as "matter"—can never be recognized as subjects except within, and on the terms of, the colonialist-capitalist subject of the bildungsroman and human rights, or on the terms of the subject that, as I have argued (Jolly 2010), is speakable, as opposed to the unspeakable subject, or as opposed to the being that is effluent community. Instead of recognition of rights, then, Oliver argues for a mode of bearing witness to the other that she terms "affirmation," not recognition, the point being that one can affirm what one cannot fully recognize; one can affirm what one *does not know,* thereby taking the kind of risk altogether foreign to the bubble, venturing onto ground that is not protected by the contract, and where one does not know whether one will be protected, and even more radically, where one can question whether protection provided by (the myth of) the bubble is even a good thing.

Within the cult of the individualism of the bildungsroman subject, who is also the official subject of certain democracies, such as that of the United

States, affirming what one does not know would be regarded as a potential source of threat. However, effluent communities see affirmation of the unknown differently, or as Lindanathi puts it in *The Reactive*, "there was no need to be fearful of everything we didn't know" (156). In this respect, the subject of the bildungsroman and human-rights regime, as Slaughter has outlined him for us, aligns with the subject who cannot affirm the other and therefore must fear the strange and attempt to turn it into the self, as colonial capitalism demands. Not only does this breed a politics of paranoia about the unknown at the national level, as has been well documented by numerous political scientists for whom this is their primary topic (Hofstadter 1964) (Knight 2002); it also breeds fear of the unknown on an individual level. However, we need to continue to remember that, within this framework, both the individual subject and the "other" objects that it fears are fictions, otherwise we risk naturalizing both the individual subject and those "it" fears as real, in the mistaken sense of ontologically unable to be reconceived or recreated. Here we can begin to understand the persistence of effluent communities as residing not in adherence to a form of subjectivity alternative to that of the bildungsroman, but in a radical and ongoing understanding of subjects as fictional, and therefore always already available for reconstruction and recreation, despite the myth of the originary or fixed subject perpetrated by other agents of structural violence, such as the state, colonialism, capitalism, racism, and as I argue in chapter 1, the human-rights regimes, in their adherence to the notion of human rights as proper to the anthropocentric subject. To put it a different way, the effluent community does *not* outsource responsibility for subject-making to the institutionalized forms of structural violence that normalize vulnerability for the marginal and security for the propertied in the Butlerian sense, under liberal structures of recognition.

Before I move to a discussion of the vexed question of resilience and how it fares under liberal regimes of recognition as opposed to risk-taking structures of affirmation, let me engage with the promised comparative reading of *Heat and Light* and *The Reactive*, in which *Heat and Light* performs the bubble, and thus enables us to see it for what it is, as the protagonist of *The Reactive* indeed does. If *Heat and Light* points to the violence of the bubble, *The Reactive* suggests ways of living that deliberately discount its myth; that is to say, *The Reactive* can be read as just one manifesto of effluent life, but a significant one nonetheless.

Heat and Light and *The Reactive*: A North–South Comparison of Economies of Extraction and Addiction

Haigh's *Heat and Light* rigorously and relentlessly describes the war, rather than the violently presupposed alignment, between the cult of the individual and the struggle for a "better life" in her description of Bakerton, a Pennsylvania town engaged in the intergenerational tradition of depending on the boom and bust of extractive industries for income. Pennsylvania has a long history of exploitation of the land for material goods that coincides with white colonization: first logging by setters, then the first oil well ever drilled in the world, then strip mining, and most recently fracking, or hydraulic fracturing, in which vertical, or more often horizontal, drilling is combined with the propulsion of liquid into the fractures to keep the oil welling up from shale.[2] Haigh's novel is tellingly bookended by two rare references to the Indigenous peoples of Pennsylvania. At the beginning of the novel, the unnamed narrator points out that the oldest person in Bakerton, Ada Thibodeaux, came from a family "two counties over, what had been Seneca land, given to Chief Cornplanter by the Commonwealth of Pennsylvania, until the state changed its mind and took it back again" (3). This colonial history does not reappear until the close of the novel, when fracking has come and appears to be going, at least from Bakerton. One of the protagonists, Rich Devlin, fantasizes about a virtually unimaginable world in which the land is still precolonial, populated by "Indians" (427). This protovision is inspired, unsurprisingly, by a TV commercial, a scene to which I shall return presently.

In between these two bookends, the mouse trap is painstakingly outlined as a series of constraining bubbles, constituted by the structural violence of colonial capitalism's ruling premises, including its naturalization of these premises as ontological or inevitable, and fixed. The subject of capitalism is itself problematic, in that the very use of "it," I admit, replicates the primary fiction of capitalism: it presents itself as an "incontrovertible realism," but is rooted in fiction. According to Emile Benveniste, the pronoun appears to be fixed but is in fact a shifting signifier, one whose meaning is as unavailable for firm identification in inverse proportion to the ways in which the fantasy of capitalism represents itself as commonsensical, transparent, normative, and inevitable: "real" (1971, 227). As Ericka Beckman writes:

Slavoj Žižek, Alain Badiou, and Mark Fisher have all argued that capitalism today presents itself as an incontrovertible source of "realism," to which there is no viable alternative. The powerful sense of realism that capitalism evokes is in a strong sense, however, rooted in fiction. As Susan Bruce and Valeria Wagner have written, in reference to the work of Cornelius Castoriadis, "the economy is the domain of capitalist societies in which the imaginary reigns most completely and most unquestioned, presenting itself as the rationale for the entire society but itself bordering on a 'systemic delirium.'" (2012, 146)

The term "capitalist societies" requires nuancing in the context of this comparison with reference to the WReC's theory of combined and uneven development.

While the developed capitalism of the United States is able to present itself as natural, inevitable, "real," the characters of Ntshanga's *The Reactive* understand capitalism as a fiction. They don't deny its effects on their lives, but neither do they accept its inevitability. Thus, while the characters of *Heat and Light* constantly represent themselves in the binary terms of winners and losers, perpetrators and victims in a game in which material goods are seen as a realm of the zero-sum game par excellence, Ntshanga's central protagonists understand that their desires and actions and very being are co-constituted through a negotiation between structural factors not within their control and their interrelations with one another. This notion of community as a subject—as opposed to the individual as the subject who wins or loses against rules set by someone or something else—creates a resilience. At the risk of exploiting puns extravagantly, if *Heat and Light* is about reactors as subjects, it is also about subjects as reactors, and *The Reactive*, while referring to those who test positive for HIV, is also referring to subjects-as-reactives.

The first sentence of *The Reactive* makes a statement that initially reads as though the narrator, Lindanathi, has assigned some men to kill his brother: "Ten years ago I helped a handful of men take my little brother's life" (3). The opening sentence is a stark intertextual reference to *Nervous Conditions*, Tsitsi Dangarembga's now classic coming-of-age story of a female protagonist, Tambudzai, who states at the beginning of that novel that she is "not sorry that my brother died" (1989, 1). Tambudzai refers to the fact that she would not have been afforded a (colonial) education if her brother had not died, owing to the primacy of male children in the distribution of meager family resources (although the older Tambudzai does come to question the violence of the colonial education she delights in as a youngster). In stark contrast, Lindanathi feels responsible for the death of his brother, as they had agreed to undertake the Xhosa initiation ceremony, that of ceremonial circumcision, into manhood together. Luthando, Lindanathi's brother, has a botched circumcision and dies two days before he is due to come out of the seclusion that circumcision initiates traditionally undertake. Lindanathi takes responsibility for this death because he fled from the ritual, leaving his brother, Luthando, as Lindanathi understands it, at risk.

While Slaughter reads Dangarembga's novel as a classic type of how postcolonial writers exploit the bildungsroman to claim human rights, this reading downplays the failure of such rights in relation to the protagonist's (Tambudzai's) cousin Nyasha, for whom the aforementioned colonial education granted her by her father, a missionary school pastor-headmaster, is fatally toxic. However, this is not territory (re)covered by Ntshange, as Lindanathi firmly tells us that the novel "isn't a story about me and my brother from the Transkei, about the Mda boys from eMthata or the village of Qokolweni, where my grandmother's bones lie polished and buried next to her Ma's. Instead I want to tell you about what happened to me in Cape Town after Luthando had taken his death" (4). Here Luthando actively "takes" his death, rather than dies, as he takes up a position with the ancestors through the ceremonies of the funeral. Further, it is significant that this novel does not oppose tradition to colonial or postcolonial modernity à la *Nervous Conditions*: the novel is about communal forms of responsibility, not the binary of the early Dangarembga novel.

The person who doesn't "take up" Luthando's death, who cannot come to terms with his responsibility in it, is Lindanathi, who subsequently, in his capacity as a lab technician, infects himself with HIV. However, the cult of individual responsibility as either perpetrator or victim does not play out in this novel. Despite the fantasies of Lindanathi and his friends Cissie and Ruan about his (Lindinathi's) dying year, which they call affectionately his "Last Life" (17), and which he thinks about less and less once he moves to Dunoon,[3] he is not a victim of HIV in the traditional sense. Indeed, it is precisely because Lindanathi perceives that he cannot react appropriately to his brother's call for companionship in the circumcision ritual that he infects himself:

One year after I graduated from tech, and a week before the sixth anniversary of LT's death, I infected myself with HIV in the laboratories. That's how I became a reactive. I never had the reactions I needed for myself, and I couldn't react when Luthando called me for help, so I gave my own body something it couldn't flee from. (141)

Unlike the selfishness of the majority of the characters in Haigh's *Heat and Light* (with the exception of the nurse Rena), Lindanathi listens when Cissie explains his weakness to him. He states: "One of the biggest problems she has with me, she says, is that I never pay enough attention to people. Every time I offer someone a shoulder to cry on, Cissie says, my biggest concern is the snot left drying on my shirt. I've told her how I think that's good, how she's phrased that" (13). Of course, the inversion in the last sentence enables the reader to think for a second that Lindanathi thinks it's good for him to be self-centered; but instead, it's the match between the aesthetics and meaning of her statement about his selfishness he likes; his affirmation is of his own "snottiness." Preceding this exchange, we discover that Lindanathi tries to make up for his lack of responsiveness with physical affection. When Cissie burns her finger cooking up the glue the trio uses to make their posters advertising that they sell the antiretrovirals that prevent HIV from developing into AIDS, Lindanathi comforts her in a way so intimate that it entirely exceeds his later mechanistic description of his sexual exploits with a pair of prostitutes he hires to make up a trio:

> ... with everything silent and her flat feeling like an old tomb around us, I bent down to touch her on the part of her finger that was dying. With her eyes still closed, Cissie raised her hand and stuck the burnt finger inside my mouth, and, sliding it slowly over my tongue, told me to suck on the skin till it came back to life.
> So I did that.
> I didn't mind doing it, either. (13)

Cissie tells Lindanathi he checks the time a lot when people are telling him their problems: "In response, I told her I'd work on it. Then I looked at my wristwatch. I guess I'm still working in it." (14).

Unlike Lindanathi, the logic that binds the characters of *Heat and Light*, with the aforementioned exception of Rena, is one of self-promotion through the exploitation of others and a deep assumption, so deep as to remain unstated, that not only material goods, but even sympathy and empathy, like that Lindanathi seeks from within himself, are commodities in a zero-sum game of human interactions. What this leads to is an array of addictions that would baffle Lauren Berlant herself, whose theory of "cruel optimism" (2011) I shall explore later in this chapter. There is the addiction of the Pennsylvanian communities and Americans at large to fossil fuels, an addiction that constructs the boom-and-bust economy of Pennsylvania, based as it is primarily on fossil fuels: "Rural Pennsylvania doesn't fascinate the world, not generally," the narrator of *Heat and Light* tells us, "but cyclically, periodically, its innards are of interest. Bore it, strip it, set it on fire, a burnt offering to the collective need" (11). This resource is seen as a preordained trap, not a set of substances whose usage can be conceived of in any way other than their exploitation, and that of the workers whose "fate" it is to mine the goods:

> More than most places, Pennsylvania is what lies beneath. Accidents of geology, larger than history, older than scripture: continents colliding, seas encroaching and receding, peat bogs incubating their treasures like a vast subterranean kiln. In the time before recorded time, Pennsylvania was booby-trapped. Blame the gods for what lies beneath, the old pagan gods, discredited now, vaguely disreputable, the unwashed old men who struck a backroom deal before Jesus was invented. (426)

The odd corollary of this, despite the cycles of the boom-and-bust economy, is that it builds in the citizens not skepticism, but faith in "the next big thing": faith in the colonialist-capitalist bubble. This faith benefits Bobby Frame, the salesman from the felicitously named Dark Elephant fracking company, which is looking to acquire drilling rights on the townsfolk's land. Further, the faith in the next big boom is associated by the narrator with the faith of the townsfolk, who the narrator implies invented Jesus themselves and proceeded to have faith in him, just as they do in the (idea of) prosperity:

> [The] past [of Bakerton] holds no interest for Bobby Frame, though he owes his success to it—distant memory of boom times,

the ghost of prosperity that lingers in the town. Here promises are met without skepticism. The landowners are churchgoers, people of faith. The agnostics—there are a few—need only to look to history: Bakerton has been favored before, tapped by Industry's magic wand. (12)

The agnostics here are not so much those that don't go to church—Rich Devlin, for example, prefers to fish, despite his belief both in the fracking promise offered by Bobby Frame and his wife and daughter's Sunday church attendance—but those few residents who refuse Bobby's offer: the lesbian couple Rena and Mack, and Con Krug, "a known crack pot. . . . A man of complicated opinions, paranoid theories that require much explaining on Open Mike, the local radio's call-in show. . . . The sort of eccentric who gets stranger with age, and he's been old as long as Rich can remember" (75). The faith about which the narrator speaks, then, is faith in capitalism. And (faith in) capitalism requires denial of the historical crises it produces.

Beckman quotes Terry Eagleton in this regard: "Capitalism is incapable of inventing a future that does not ritualistically reproduce its present," and further, she adds, "capitalism is incapable of creating a vision of the past that does not reinforce its resolute presentism" (2012, 147). Following in this vein, Beckman argues for a privileging of fiction as that which can read the recurring catastrophes in capitalist history without glossing over them: "If we accept that history under capitalism is not one of linear progress but instead one of repetition, reversal, and ruin, literary works of the past can provide a window onto the repetitive and cyclical logic of capital that continues to mark our present" (148). Neither *Heat and Light* nor *The Reactive*, both published in 2016, can be considered literary works of the past. But they nevertheless show how the "the imaginative and indeed fictive" underpinnings of capitalism come to light in what Beckman terms the "throes of crisis" (148).

Beckman remarks on fictions from South America, from countries she discusses as accorded a place in, borrowing from Dipesh Chakrabarty, "the waiting room of history," following the teleologies of modernity and development, at best "emerging," sometimes simply "underdeveloped," but sometimes distinctly "backward." But the postcolonial residents of the South Africa of *The Reactive*, I argue forcefully, understand themselves to be living in perpetual crisis and have little or no faith in "the next best thing": they are not interested in entering "the waiting room" because they know the colonialist-capitalist prize to be a swindle. Conversely, *Heat and Light* demonstrates relentlessly what I experience as the airlessness of a culture in which those who question capitalism are considered both unspeakable and in turn to be the ranters of the insane, à la Butler: like Con Krug, they are considered deeply eccentric and positively obstructionist. In this sense, the community of *The Reactive* is in some way inoculated against, or resilient in the face of, the faith in capitalism held by the majority of Bakerton's residents. This is not to say that Lindanathi and his friends deny the material comforts of life, or even the use of so-called recreational drugs, as we shall see; but their faith in them is limited, just as their demonization of them is equally limited.

This is a comparison I explore through the metonymical relation of addiction to capitalism. In *Heat and Light,* addiction is portrayed as a normalized relation to all resources, human and material, and in fact, the rhetorical gambit of the novel could be described as representing capitalism so realistically, so seamlessly, that capitalism's artificiality is highlighted by the Teflon description of it: nothing will stick to it, just as it doesn't stick to itself.

On the other hand, capitalized instrumentalization is seen as having its limits for human well-being in *The Reactive*. I am not making a moral argument against drug use. I argue, instead, that highly "developed" capitalist countries like the United States relate to all resources through a dominant model of addiction, without recognition that, while they may label as "addiction" only the pattern of chemical dependency on illegal drugs, still other patterns such as "workaholism" and certain relations to foods and to others' attention may also be classified as addiction, including the culture's primordial respect for extractive industries.

Before I discuss scenes of addiction and drug use in both novels, however, it makes sense to point out that South Africa is also "what lies beneath it," from gold to platinum to diamonds and back. It is the world's largest producer of chrome, manganese, platinum, vanadium, and vermiculite. It is the second largest producer of ilmenite, palladium, rutile, and zirconium. It is also the world's third largest coal exporter. South Africa is also a huge producer of iron ore; in 2012, it overtook India to become the world's third biggest iron ore supplier to China, which is the world's largest consumers of iron ore. It lacks only oil, but it converts its abundant low-grade lignite coal into oil to offset some of this need. Its history of colonial rule, followed by the apartheid regime and collusion with capitalism, have ensured that the benefits of these resources have been profoundly inequitably distributed. Indeed, the resources on occasion ensured that the apartheid regime was upheld. Margaret Thatcher and Ronald Reagan in the 1980s, for example, supported apartheid vigorously, since they feared the fall of such resources into the hands of both the "Black" (majority population) and "Red" (communist) "perils."

The exploitation of highly policed, Black, migrant labor forces, from Rhodes's controlling development of the diamond mines in Kimberly to the so-called hostels of the Witwatersrand goldfields, has at least one positive outcome: the notion that such labor will at some point be of benefit to the laborer, never believed by the laborers themselves, was explicitly denied even by Hendrik Verwoerd, in his role as Minister of Bantu Affairs in 1954, before he became Prime Minister of the Republic in 1958.[4] The National Union of Mineworkers, who never held such an illusion in apartheid days, was a huge factor in the African National Congress victory against apartheid in 1994; and the police shootings of mineworkers at Lonmin platinum mine in 2012 in the postapartheid era bear witness to the ongoing history of mineworker abuse and exploitation.[5] Indeed, the history of mining in South Africa is simultaneously the history of the violent and deliberate disintegration of Black families over the colonial and apartheid periods, and the concentration of ownership among elites who determine stock market values. This legacy, entrenched by President Thabo Mbeki's liberal economic policies, will have effects for the century yet to come.

If the United States is among the global leaders in an addiction to fossil fuels, Haigh constructs this addiction not as exceptional, but as part and parcel of colonial capitalism's entrenchment of patterns of addiction as the normalized human approach to all resources, material and other. This is particularly true, in the world of *Heat and Light,* of how one garners attention for *oneself.* Wesley Peacock, as a child, loves being at home with his mother, rather than at school, and fantasizes about being the boy in the eponymous bubble of the movie. Here the bubble is seen as protective, not constricting, and creates risk reduction in the mind of the obsessed Wesley, later to become Pastor Wes. Ironically, it is precisely because his mother refuses to leave the bubble of her house in the proximity of the Three Mile

Island core meltdown that, he believes, he later develops the cancer that kills him. In his reflections after his death, which form the only part of the narrative from the perspective of the afterlife and its only unrealistic aspect, he muses that he contained his wife, Pastor Jess, in too much of a bubble that involved just the two of them. The attention he needed made introducing a child into the family impossible. The suggestion that Wes can see the bubble for what it is only after his death suggests that a certain kind of character cannot exist within the bubble. It's not only that an effluent subject is not admitted to the bubble because the effluent subject is not recognized; it's also that an effluent subject would be stifled, unable to thrive, within the bubble.

An addiction to attention is also played out in the life of Shelby Devlin, now married to Rich, the brother who bought the farm from his brothers and plans to run it as a farm again, once he has garnered enough money from working as a prison guard—he is placing all his eggs in the capitalist bubble, as his name indicates. Shelby's sister dies of lupus as a child, at which point Shelby grabs the attention that her sister has held as "the sick one" and thrives on the attention now given to her by Pastor Wes, as the surviving sister. Rich Devlin is attracted to her because he thinks he can control her. Ultimately, though, it is she who forces them to abandon the old farmhouse and move into a prefab on the same property, owing to what she experiences as a mold allergy. (She is the first to point out that the fracking Rich agrees to in order to fund his farming dream is poisoning the water.) Most sinister, however, is her control of her daughter Olivia's life. Olivia has constant stomach ailments, which Shelby claims prove her child is taking after her own frail health. Inquiries by Rena the nurse into Olivia's health, on the suspicion that the child is negatively affected by fracking, turn up the specialist's suggestion, not provable but hideously present nevertheless, that Shelby is feeding ipecac to her child, thus creating Olivia's illness through Munchausen's syndrome by proxy. This is borne out by the narrative, as elsewhere in the text Rich claims his car constantly smells of the candy-grape scent of Olivia's illness, which is indeed the smell of ipecac. This notion of an emotional zero-sum economy of attention from others implies that Shelby understands that the only way she can continue to get attention is through her own, or her child's, ill-being. Hence, she visits Pastor Jess for counseling, jealously guarding her time with the Pastor and eventually writing a note to Jess anonymously to inform Jess that Herc, the fracking-employed boyfriend Pastor Jess takes up with after Wes's death from cancer, is married. This addiction to ill health as a means of gaining affection reaches its comic-tragic zenith just before Wes's death when Shelby, bringing him food, attempts to have sex with him. At first, he is willing, but then he shies away. Initially they kiss with abandon, as he is said to "step out of his *bubble*, into the very short future, . . . abandoning hope, honor, the illusion of consequence" (314; emphasis added). What he sees as Shelby's "truly exotic" nature because she is "willing to lie down with a dead man" is, in fact, the logical conclusion of Shelby's repeated pattern of behavior: searching for attention through associating herself with illness, and in this case, with Death personified.

This scene of garnering attention through illness is parodied by the depiction of the drug- and HIV-counseling culture in *The Reactive*. Cissie, Ruan, and our narrator, Lindanathi, regularly use drugs, but they attend the meetings to garner clients. Lindanathi, as an insured HIV-positive individual, receives his antiretroviral (ARV) drugs as long as he passes on CD4 counts (counts of the viral load in his blood) to his caseworker. He is shoddy in complying with this demand because, rather than take his ARVs regularly, he sells them at great profit to those without access to ARVs, either because they are not insured or because they prefer to purchase the drugs rather than "come out" through an official diagnosis, or both. This was a lucrative industry prior to the Constitutional Court–mandated public provision of ARVs in South Africa in 2003. What is not skeptical, however, is Lindanathi's observation that, "like most places filled with the sick and the dying, there's always an opportunity to learn something about being a person here" (33). While Shelby in *Heat and Light* sees illness as a place for herself to suck up affection like a never-ending sponge, Lindanathi has an entirely different experience with a woman at "group" called Olive, two vowels away from Shelby's daughter Olivia, felicitously enough for the purpose of this comparison.

Olive's concern is that her drug addiction has made her son Emile lose all respect for her: "Today, she shares her latest suspicions about Emile. Olive says her apologies have started to harden him, to make him believe she is a woman who deserves nothing better than scorn. Listening to her, the rest of us nod" (35). It becomes clear, however, that this nod, at least on Lindanathi's part, is not in agreement with her son, but in acknowledgment of her shame. Unlike Shelby, Lindanathi is very aware of the limits of the value of his sympathy for Olive. He is not unsympathetic, but realizes, with a non-selfishness totally foreign to Shelby, that he cannot help Olive; and further, drowning himself in her life becomes an excuse for him to avoid responsibility for his own actions, growth, and happiness:

> Olive's the one I've come to feel the most for in our meetings, but there's nothing I can do to help. She suffers from something I have no treatment for, and I can only watch her when she drops her head in shame. Often, I've had to avert my eyes when Olive starts to weep, but today my gaze remains passive and arrested on her frame, I realize my feelings for her have been drained from me, and that I can no longer use her as a hiding place. (35)

On one level, of course, Lindanathi's statement that he has nothing that can cure Olive means that his ARVs can't fix her addiction; on another, it suggests first that the lack of self-respect she feels is not remediable by drugs, medical or recreational, and second that Lindanathi himself still has to reckon with his own shame, that of abandoning his brother. If Shelby uses others' illnesses as her comfort in one way or another, Lindanathi assumes responsibility to give up this flight from responsibility for the self.

Further, he is aware of the limits of the culture of confession imposed by counseling-group mores. While Lindanathi takes what is said by the group members respectfully, he simultaneously knows it's not the whole story: survival of this effluent community means keeping to yourself some of the story; otherwise, one risks complete colonization, as it were, by those seeking your "full confession." And they are not the ones who have to go back into quotidian life having bared their souls merely for the sake of "talking therapy." Resilience under such circumstances looks like this:

> In most meetings, half the members don't make the move to draw close to one another. We enter each session prepared to deflect the counsel leader, whose job is to put whatever remains of us under glass. If you listen to counselors, they tell you they want full disclosure in meetings, but most of us know to hand out the facts in small doses only. Therapy won't walk you home after you pack up the chairs. Telling too much about yourself can leave you feeling broken into, as if your head were a conquered city offered to the

group for pillaging. This how we know Olive won't finish Emile's story in front of us. I close my eyes again. (35)

The conquered city of the simile is the city of Cape Town, the primary setting of the novel, and a reference to its deeply colonized past and present. Of all the big cities of South Africa, Cape Town, in part due to its unique geography, remains the most divided city in terms of racial segregation through physical settlement. It was also the nexus of the trade that included slaves as goods in southern Africa, exported elsewhere across the oceans, or kept by the colonizers in the Cape white settlements. Both Cape Town and Lindanathi exceed their recognition as zones of historical shame. When Lindanathi closes his eyes, he is not shutting out Olive, but recognizing that he cannot *be* Olive, that he is not reduced to witnessing the spectacle of her shame, and that his inward gaze will protect him from living through the emotional lives of others, the latter being the practice to which Shelby is addicted.

There is also an awareness in *The Reactive* of the danger money brings, and what it can and can't do. At one point a mysterious man offers Lindanathi and his friends more than they can imagine for a supply of ARVs. It turns out that the man, who is masked because his face is deeply scarred, does not want ARVs at all: he wants to give his daughter, who lives in the same block as the three friends, money and a Canadian passport to offer her a future better than the one she spends with her aunt in Cape Town. He is clearly a person who lives beyond or outside the law, and he does indeed deposit money into the three friends' accounts after they deliver the money and passport to his daughter, whom he cannot have contact with for her own safety. Before they agree to undertake the transaction, however, Lindanathi, Ruan, and Cissie worry about the danger of being caught by the police; and Lindanathi and Ruan worry about taking Cissie to the neighborhood where the deal is to take place, as being a woman makes her vulnerable to sexual assault. Nevertheless, they agree they want the money and fantasize about retiring to the country to grow dope, just as Rich fantasizes about returning the farm to farming. In the end, however, it turns out that the money is withdrawn from their accounts, probably because of South Africa's highly restricted currency, in which banks monitor large deposits for money laundering and other forms of fraud. But this disappointment is mentioned merely as a happenstance, not as a deep tragedy.

By contrast, money is the future, especially for Rich Devlin and his father. Darren, Rich's brother, spoils his future with a drug habit that uses up his scholarship and the money his family gets together for him to study science at Johns Hopkins. By the time we meet him, he is a counselor at a rehab center who staves off his addiction to drugs by spending every possible moment at the center—he has redirected drugaholism into workaholism. When he is forced to take his mandated accumulated holiday, he reluctantly goes back to Bakerton. Here he helps out his father and brother in the bar owned by the family, and has a brief affair with the waitress, Gina, who is herself addicted to crack. He finally returns early to the city, knowing he will start using again in the environment of the bar.

Herein lies a complicated irony: Dick Devlin, Rich and Darren's father, a former miner, is considered a success story as an ex-miner. He has fulfilled his dream and bought a bar, financed by his brother's money left to him, accumulated through payments for black lung disease. Dick himself is able to lend money to Rich when Rich buys out his siblings to own the farm outright, as he finally has some money accumulated from his own payments for black lung. Thus, the destruction of one's body is compensated for in money that feeds one's dreams, and success is determined by having a fatal disease. Dick is considered a success because he works at this bar, while the other retired miners drink each day at the Legion, waiting for death to come to them. Rich signs the lease to Dark Elephant to enable drilling on his property to fulfill his dream of farming his father's land with dairy cattle. First, he is forced to move from the old farmhouse owing to Shelby's mold allergy; then he ends up shipping in water because the fracking has contaminated his well. Finally, he realizes that he will never fulfill his dream: he can't even go for second best, selling the family farm and buying another one, as Dark Elephant hasn't paid the companies it contracts to frack his land, and their claim to unpaid fees is represented by a lien against the farm: he cannot therefore sell his own land.

The comparison made by the narrator, focalized through Rich's reflections in the closing section of the work, is stark: "Who had been the bigger fool, Rich or Devlin, was impossible to say" (426). The relation of capitalism to the body that becomes visible in the Devlins' collective narrative is that the body itself is an extractive zone: the body is traded for a supposed capitalist gain that never materializes, or if it does, is never quite worth the loss of wellness paid for the ever decreasing and receding prize. This prize, for the ironically named Rich, as in the case of his father Dick, is now also a settlement: a settlement for damages to the farm environment that can never be reversed, just as the damage the loss of his dream does to Rich can never be reversed: "He will never be a farmer. When his settlement comes—if it comes—he could, in theory, buy another farm. The point was to work this land—Pap's land, bought and paid for by [Rich's] own hard labor, ten years of overtime at Deer Run" (426). Hard labor here is a pun, as Rich works at the prison called Deer Run. At first, he was attracted to law enforcement by the idea of the noble law-keeper; now he understands that being a prison warder simply means cleaning up society's messes, the ones everyone else leaves behind. Darren's drug addiction does not leave him much worse off than his brother. In addition to this, Darren's addiction puts in high relief the fact that addiction is not the antipathy to capitalism, but its modus operandi. Indeed, it is Darren's very experience of addiction that renders him able to work as a counselor at the rehab center. It's made clear in the text that all he does is transfer his addiction from drugs to work at the rehab center.

In contrast, Lindanathi stops feeding off the exploitation of his own body when he quits selling his ARVs. He moves back to Bhut' Vuyo's home in Dunoon, a shipping container in which Bhut' Vuyo and his family live. Bhut' Vuyo is whom he stayed with after his mother couldn't bear having him at home after the death of his younger brother, Luthando. Bhut' Vuyo begs Lindanathi to come home to Dunoon and finally get circumcised, and Lindanathi puts this off for as long as he can, even trying to fend off Bhut' Vuyo's pleas with money, which he knows will offend the man: Bhut' Vuyo cannot be bought off or bought out.

When he does return to Dunoon, Lindanathi helps Bhut' Vuyo rebuild the long-drop toilet, which Bhut' Vuyo builds in defiance of the government-provided chemical toilets (portaloos), whose active ingredients have long stopped working. While Lindanathi understands that this is a political project of Bhut Vuyo's, so as not to be (or be seen to be) dependent on the government for the pathetic toilets offered in mitigation for "informal settlements" where actual plumbing has never been installed, Lindanathi takes part in the effort wholeheartedly. Neither the portaloos provided by the municipality nor the long-drop they build works particularly well, but the point is the labor and its gesture, which are in excess of practical instrumentalization.

By rejecting an absolute logic of instrumentalization, of his own and others' bodies not least, Lindanathi breaks the metonymical relation between capitalism and the body. It also becomes clear that he has always understood that a metaphorical relation between capitalism and human relations does not exist within the bubble, as such metaphorization would elide the cooption of bodies by capitalism as both the means and objects of extractive industry, means in terms of labor and objects in terms of sexual assault, exploitation, and organ harvesting as commercial exchange. Built into Lindanathi's narrative is a warning to the reader of *The Reactive* against following the counselor's diagnostic reading, a warning not to read the addicts/HIV-positives as victims or objects of diagnostic recognition or to allow the professional counselor to "offer" a reading of the "victim"-sufferer that empowers transition back into the fold of the bubble. First, one cannot depend upon a narrative of full confession for one's knowledge as a reader; second, one cannot develop a paternalistic approach to a sufferer such as Olive without using this to escape one's own challenges and/or feed one's own ego; and third, as if demonstrative of the first two cautions to the reader, the participants may hold within them elements of resilience of which the reader or the participants themselves may be completely unaware.[6] In *The Reactive*, unlike *Heat and Light*, the mouse may have ways of escaping the mousetrap now and then; and these moments of freedom are—paradoxically, from the perspective of "the land of the free"—garnered through relinquishment of the logic of instrumentalism and accumulation, the very promise of the game of the mousetrap.

When Lindanathi returns to Dunoon, he both is circumcised and takes a job at a spaza shop, an informal shack shop that sells food staples, cellphone time, cigarettes, and other such commodities. He lives with Bhut' Vuyo's family, knowing, as Bhut' Vuyo warns him, that the family is not wealthy: in fact, it is poor. The same newspapers Bhut' Vuyo and Lindanathi use to "wallpaper" the inside of the container, Lindanathi wrinkles in his hands to soften before using as toilet paper. Further, the bars of Sunlight soap (a brand known to all across sub-Saharan Africa as economical: the long bar can be cut into blocks for individual use), which are a step up from washing powder, are reserved for washing the body, while the powder is used for hands. Lindanathi has actually "dropped" his "living standard" considerably by moving from inner-city Cape Town back to Dunoon. There is no going to restaurants or drinking wine; he curtails his endless string of substance abuse, although he still sniffs glue and smokes cigarettes. He meets a girlfriend, whose skin he reminisces about in ways completely different from his use of the aforementioned sex workers; and he understands the community has taken him in, just as they take in others who may even be their enemies. But the "taking in" is not the same as a biblical turning of the other cheek, as we shall see.

One morning Lindanathi is on his way to work at the spaza shop when he sees unrest on the street. He quickly surmises that this is not one of the ubiquitous strikes. Ominously, tires are burning at the scene. In earlier novels and Truth and Reconciliation Commission testimony, this would more than likely indicate a so-called "necklacing," in which a township community would place burning tires around a Black person suspected of acting as an undercover agent for the apartheid government. Here, however, it transpires that the youth has tried to take in the pensioners of the community with a pyramid scheme, defrauding them of their money; and, when he is challenged, in a mad act of aggression, he tries to burn the community down, and hence the burning tires. The men of the community, not much older than the youth, drive a shopping trolley over him but are advised by the women not to beat him up too hard and to dress him when they're done, as his only garb is a green vest, apparently stolen from the clothesline nearby. In a strange coincidence, the young man, whom we later learn is named Siseko, yells that a faceless man will come and the community will then be free, an apparent reference to the masked man of the earlier mystery. The women of the community recognize him as a madman, *ligeza eli*, and the community does indeed dress him and subsequently take him in, in the reverse of the way he earlier "took in" its pensioners.

Later, Lindanathi sketches the man with the damaged face who got him, Cissie, and Ruan to deliver money and a passport to his daughter, Ethelia. Siseko recognizes the usually masked face as that of the faceless man he has been prophesying will save the community. In this respect, the women of the community recognize as a madman the youth who suggests that the man who makes money off others will come to save them, playing the prophet of that ultimate pyramid scheme, capitalism, *but* a madman to be pitied, not demonized. And Lindanathi himself refuses to demonize the man in the mask, whom Lindanathi has long since nicknamed Ambroise Paré, after he heard of the so-called headless man of Paré, the first man who developed prostheses to assist men wounded in battle.[7] "To me," Lindanathi tells us, "Monsieur Paré had only been a parent, and Ethelia his daughter: a father" (156). Siseko walks away with the picture of the mask.

At this point, the defaced visage and the mask of the man have become indistinguishable in Lindanathi's narrative, since we do not know whether he has drawn the "faceless man," as Siseko calls him, or "the mask" Siseko is said to have carried off, which is the subject of the sketch Lindanathi made. However, it appears, what the mask may hide, and indeed the mask itself, is not only not to be feared, but also to be regarded as a reminder of the respect debility commands:

> We [Lindanathi and Siseko] smoked in silence after that, and I remember feeling a sense of peace rushing into me as I watched him walking away with the mask. I knew I wouldn't be the only one to do him a favor that day, to make sure he sometimes landed on his feet. The community had taken him in, like it had done with me, and there was no need to be fearful of anything we didn't know. (157)

This is, among other interpretations, a parody of a deformed crook claimed as a potential savior for his exploitative practices yet revealed to be (merely) a father. This domestication in the place of demonization prevents capital, which is metonymically indistinguishable from its mask, from becoming a rampant symbol. Rather than capitalism harbingering the prophet/profit, as it desires to be seen doing, its own greatest myth is revealed: that progress, meaning movement into the field of global capital relations, is undermined as both inevitable and desirable, bringing down with it the notion of capitalism as a subject mystically divorced from human machinations. Peace comes to Lindanathi, the peace so markedly absent from *Heat and Light*, through a negotiation with the future that relinquishes absolute control of the individual: "There was no need to be fearful of anything we didn't know" is an enunciation of the reverse of the desire to be, and remain, the boy in the bubble (57).

The South African state starts to provide ARVs free of charge and Lindanathi stays on his medication: he also finally gets tested. It turns out that the virus "is arrested in his blood" (156). He is what is known as a slow progressor, or as he puts it, slow to react. His name, Lindanathi, is a girl's name taken from the daughter of a friend of his mother who works overtime at a factory to get money for her girl-child's education (perhaps yet another intertextual reference to Dangarembga's *Nervous Conditions*, in which Tambudzai's education depends on her brother's death; here, in contrast, the mother seeks to educate her girl-child). Unlike the active principle of *doing* that characterizes the settler-colonial economy, the injunction of Lindanathi's name is *to wait*. The name means "Wait with us," and it transpires that this is the promise he has made to Bhut' Vuyo and his Dunoon community: to wait with them. The question "for what?" is not the point; the point is to go through, with the community, whatever life next presents them. Unlike the narrative trajectory of *Heat and Light*, then, the point is not the consistent deferral of an individual's dreams from within the unsustainable boom-and-bust economy, but an actual practice of *waiting-with* in which community resources, material and otherwise, are not envisioned as the basis of a zero-sum game, with winners and losers. The so-called faceless man, nicknamed Ambroise Paré by Lindanathi, is not a winner, but simply a father; and Lindanathi is not a loser, but a community member who loves and is loved back, in turn.

None of this is to deny the privations of poverty, but it is to suggest that getting out of poverty is not always the primary driver of a community's ways of being in the decolonial world. At the beginning of *Heat and Light*, as I noted earlier, comes the first mention of the Indigenous inhabitants of the United States through the figure of Chief Cornplanter. At the end of the novel, Rich Devlin tries to imagine what the land would have been like without settler colonialism, his only access to such a vision being through the tawdry genre of the TV advertisement. In this reflection, we understand that, for him at least, being in the face of others having more money is an existential condition, the only thing that *matters*:

> Rich Devlin recalls, often, a famous TV commercial of his childhood: the Indian chief looking over a trash-strewn highway, a single tear sliding down his cheek—a public service agreement, designed to make people stop littering—but the ad hasn't turned him into a tree hugger, as it was clearly meant to do. It sparked, instead, his fascination with American Indians—who, he discovered, weren't the villains the old westerns had made them out to be. At nine years old, for the first and last time in his life, he read voraciously: adventure stories, encyclopedias, anything with an Indian in it. Apache, Seneca, Cherokee, Chicksaw. How he had loved those names, the cascading syllables. Reading, he imagined waking up in a teepee or a pueblo to a different life entirely, in which boys weren't forced to take spelling tests or deliver newspapers or learn catechism, the daily gauntlet of responsibility that had begun for

him and wouldn't end until he was too old to hunt or fish, too old to do anything but watch TV commercials and fall asleep in his chair. (426–27)

The catechism he learns and is repeating is a narrative of victimization through colonial capitalism, of which the religious catechism is only the metonymic part. He reflects that he learned that none of his reflections matter when he was at sea on a vast aircraft carrier sailing to the first Persian Gulf war, "a place that mattered for one reason only": oil. He and his fellow men called the carrier, the *SS Roosevelt,* the Big Stick: "When he thinks of it now, he imagines the Big Stick gliding over a vast sea of other people's money, a thought that didn't occur to him at the time." And then the novel ends: "We are all sailors" (427).

Responsibility for understanding how *not* to victimize oneself through addiction to the injunction to acquire—and acquire the right things according to the principle of mimetic desire, the things everyone else wants—is viewed very differently in *The Reactive*: avoidance of such responsibility brings restlessness, and acceptance of it brings peace, maturity, and an ability to enjoy the quotidian in life. This is not to say that one form of the experience of responsibility (the responsibility to acquire under settler capitalism or the responsibility not to victimize oneself) is more authentic than the other, although one is certainly more attached to an experience of freedom rather than of containment. Settler capitalism is a spectacularly claustrophobic space in the sphere of Haigh's mousetrap. Even if the relation between material resources and economies of feeling and affect were metaphorical in capitalism, rather than metonymical, the space between the thing itself and that which forms a metaphor of it might at least leave some breathing room. In metonymy, no such space exists; the realm is airless, filled with the material of the metonym itself.

Effluent Resilience as Persistence under Global Capitalism

This raises the question of the supposed immunity or resilience of effluent communities such as that of Bhut' Vuyo's Dunoon shantytown. The politics of immunity proposed by Esposito in his 2010 *Communitas* and 2011 *Immunitas* rests on the *unstated metaphor* of that which is extrinsic being taken in by the nation in small measure, to ward off the danger of armies marching in(to) the nation in the future. The metaphor derives from the actual medical practices of inoculation and homeopathy, although Esposito himself does not recognize these origins, in part possibly because he does not write his philosophy of community/immunity with any sense that the reader is to understand its central metaphor *as metaphor*. In the light of Esposito's theory, one could argue that Lindanathi's HIV is a figure of such a politics of immunity. However, the sheer embodiment of illness in *The Reactive*, including substance abuse, mitigates taking the body as figure, seeing this metaphorization as a violation of bodily integrity. What I want to spend some time on here, however, is not the question of a politics of immunity as resilience, but the very conceptualization of resilience within effluent communities, or what we might call decolonial persistence.

In her 2016 "Rethinking Vulnerability and Resistance," Butler has argued against *resilience* as a term that outsources responsibility for disempowerment to disadvantaged communities, what she terms "neo-liberal resilience." That is to say, she argues that framing resilience as an attribute of communities who are, relatively speaking, unable to access resources to further their own well-being, such as education, health, and environmental well-being, enables the blaming of those communities for their own victimization vis-á-vis the inequitable resources global capitalism requires and sustains (12–17). While I understand Butler's caution about relatively well-resourced communities using resilience as a way of leaving poorer communities to their own devices under the sign of resilience, I argue that Butler's caution about resilience stems from a binary that sees effluent communities as victims within a global game of monopoly. That is to say, I argue that there must be a way of conceptualizing resilience such that it neither leaves the vulnerable to their own devices, "outsourcing" responsibility for their vulnerability back to them as Butler fears, nor frames impoverished communities purely within an identity of victimhood, without *any* agency. What the comparison of *Heat and Light* with *The Reactive* seems to teach us is that, within the (non)ethics of colonial capitalism, there is no need to label those who are at the mercy of the system as victims, because they do so themselves. Remember Rich, through whom the narrative voice focalizes the thought that "who had been the bigger fool, Rich or Devlin, was impossible to say" (426).

Berlant describes this apparent self-victimization in her category of "cruel optimism," in which what one desires stands directly in the way of one's own well-being (2011). She posits cruel optimism as a relational dynamic whereby individuals remain attached to "compromised conditions of possibility" or "clusters of promises" embedded in desired object-ideas, even when the attachments inhibit the conditions for flourishing and fulfilling such promises (24, 23). Put more bluntly, "a relation of cruel optimism exists when something you desire is actually an obstacle to your flourishing" (1). She nevertheless argues, in her conceptualization of "lateral agency," that "people are neither dupes to the interests of power as such nor gods of their own intention" (105). The point is that one would have to know how the interests of power are operating in each case not to be duped by them, which creates a discipline of eternal vigilance verging on the paranoid and the assumption of an ability to know what the interests of power are and the multiple ways in which they might manifest themselves, suggesting that the interests of power are backed by a will that itself can be identified. I agree with the notion of an agency on the part of the citizen that is neither a victimized dupe nor a controlling perpetrator, the two stock figures of the cult of the individual that colonial capitalism breeds; but I disagree with Berlant's notion that lateral agency expresses itself in the self-*interruption* of the self from the overwhelming discipline of the self, or what she calls "self-maintenance" in the face of the impossible task of making the good life happen (116).

In her introduction, Berlant points out that the archive of her project is drawn from the United States and contemporary Europe, and I have no intention of accusing her of a generalizability to other contexts, such as that of the postapartheid South Africa at stake in *The Reactive*. Instead, I wish to use her work as a kind of negative outline to pose the outlines of a postcolonial resilience, or a resilience of the effluent, that we shall call "persistence." For example, Berlant argues that "food is one of the few spaces of controllable, reliable pleasure people have" (115). Maybe so in the world of which she speaks, but in areas of food insecurity, food becomes the object not only of great desire, but of anxiety about its absence, since its presence is far from reliable. Further, this is complicated by ARV regimens, which create nausea and other digestive problems if not accompanied by food. Similarly, Berlant claims that, "unlike alcohol or other drugs, food is necessary to existence, part of the care of the self, the reproduction of life" (115). Maybe so, but there are many who would feed others of their community before themselves, as the self has a different meaning in Lindanathi's lexicon. Further, for the HIV-infected, ARV drugs are indeed necessary to life, as much as food is. As Zackie Achmat, founder of the Treatment Action Campaign, demonstrated with his protest comprising a refusal to take

ARVs until they were publicly available, HIV-positive people can progress quickly to dangerously low CD4 counts and full-blown AIDS without medication; and "drug" strikes to demand appropriate HIV treatment have a venerable and substantial history in South Africa, including hunger strikes, which highlight ARVs as just as much of a necessity as food in a positive world.[8]

What then is the difference in context, and how do I construct a sense of nonexploitative resilience, or persistence, to the effluent community of which Lindanathi forms a part? Berlant's argument is that the genres of striving for the good life continue to be meaningful and essential to people's well-being long after the actual post–World War II promise of the good life is attainable in actuality for the majority. This addiction to the good life created the structural intensity of cruel optimism and manifests the structural violence of colonial capitalism's promise, and people's attachment to that promise, in the face of worsening employment opportunities and lessening remuneration. Berlant eschews the drama of trauma phrased as a singularity, and instead argues for the insistence of quotidian trauma, a nonexceptional set of circumstances that wears down the individual. Here we come to a key point, however: the promise of colonial capitalism was never *for* Indigenous peoples, as Alexis Wright's *Carpentaria*, analyzed in my final chapter, demonstrates; nor was it ever *for* the Black people of South Africa. Of course, there has been the rise of a Black middle class in the wake of Thabo Mbeki's liberal economic policies, but these are the "exactsame" (to use Haigh's word in *Heat and Light* [66, 68, 118, 412]) policies that have maintained and extended poverty among the Black majority.

The key point here is that the good life does not hold the sway it has in places where the nation-state has historically provided protection from violence, à la Butler, as the community knows the state first and foremost as a primary source of structural and actual violence, making the myth of the bubble unsustainable in colonized and Aboriginal communities. Thus, we may rewrite Butler in the case of South Africa: to be exposed to the violence wielded by the nation-state is to be forever (at best) skeptical of, and (at worst) unable to believe in, any protection proffered by the nation-state and what may be its associated capitalist practices. To bring this back to a concrete scene in *The Reactive*, we can rehearse how the counseling group has a general dislike of Neil, who, unlike the others, has had a precipitous fall from the grace of the middle class through his drug use. Instead of gaining sympathy, like Olive, he is viewed by the group as a parody of the citizen who commands the good life. In fact, precisely because he used to command the good life, had he contracted HIV rather than "just" an addiction to heroin, Lindanathi, Ruan, and Cissie could have made a lot of money off him by selling Lindanathi's ARVs to him. He would be a perfect target, vulnerable to the shame of declaring he has HIV, not on an insurance program owing to his unemployed status, and yet wealthy enough to pay for them. He isn't liked by the group precisely because he has been a good-life inhabitant:

> He's a former math teacher from a gated estate in Westlake. He's been divorced twice and has rails on both his arms, the result of a heroin habit that followed from years of blow. He taught private school for thirteen years, he says, and maybe that's why no-one likes him here. I've heard some of the older members say he won't make it through the year, and if you look at him, that isn't hard to believe. This comes from the old users, mostly. . . . They look at him and shake their heads. . . .
>   Like most addicts, Neil has an excuse for each time he feels his life is cracking open. Today, he wants a mass deportation of all the illegal immigrants in Cape Town. We should start off with the Nigerians, he tells us, and follow it up with Somalis.
>   I look over and find Cissie rolling her eyes.
>   Out of the three of us, Cissie's the one Neil bored the most. I remember how she once asked us why he didn't just get HIV already. Maybe it was an awful thing to say, but Ruan and I laughed because it was true. Even though Neil's a serf in his community, he's a nobleman in ours. We could've pulled a lot of money out of him. (32–33)

Neil's status as a nobleman is hardly desirable in this instance; in fact, it renders him vulnerable to their exploitation of him.

Now let me assay the promised comparison of Berlant's "cruel optimism," epitomized so painfully in *Heat and Light,* and postcolonial persistence, or the resilience of the effluent, as I identify it in the *The Reactive*. In cruel optimism, what you desire is an obstacle to your flourishing, whereas Lindanathi and company strongly suspect that flourishing is an impossibility, a sell job—hence their complete lack of surprise when the money from the faceless/masked man, Ambroise Paré, in exchange for their drop off to his daughter, doesn't eventuate. What is interesting, however, is that they make the drop off after they know the money has been withdrawn from their accounts, in an exchange that exceeds capitalist exchange values:

> We never hear from the ugly man again. I guess there isn't much else to say about him. He's just one of this city's many ciphers, we decide, one of the strange things that happen in the alleyways of the Southern Peninsula. . . . In any case the money is retracted from our account, laundered most likely, and he never comes back for the ARVs. To the three of us, our planned meeting with Ethelia [his daughter] takes on an inevitable air. (127)

About a week later, they hand over the package containing money and her Canadian passport to Ethelia.

Further, Berlant argues that the situation of cruel optimism obtains as a genre of social time and practice in which a relation of persons and worlds is changing; and the rules for habituation and the genres of storytelling about it are unstable. However, the instability, despite its demarcation by quotidian crisis, assumes an original stability, a background historically of a sustainable good life. But in effluent communities, storytelling genres never were about habituation to an impossible fantasy of either unshakable, protected endurance or the good life; further, the subject never mistook itself as a sovereign being, and was therefore never a sovereign individual, but intersubjectively co-constituted and animist.

Berlant's world assumes the optimism of a "slow death," or death by colonialist-capitalist attrition, whereas Lindanathi's community does not assume endurance to be more desirable than a not-so-slow death. And while Berlant's cruel optimism is definitively secular, Lindanathi's world is not. He remembers how his uncle, Bra Ishaak, cautioned him as a child for killing crabs merely for sport, "warning us that at night we would be visited by the forbears of these crabs, who would knock on our doors with bodies as tall as men" (100). Lindanathi remembers Bra Ishaak primarily as the person who instilled in him, through reference to the sea, that the natural world has no boundaries. The natural world includes death, as "when Bra Ishaak hung himself, it was . . . a Thursday morning back in Uitenhage; he wore a sailor's hat on the day he finally chose to leave us, his family, behind" (101). In this sense Bra Ishaak's choice is not suicide in the shamed sense of the act within a Western topology, nor is death the exoticized end, as it is in both *Cruel Optimism* and *Heat and Light*. In fact, the primary relation in *The Reactive* is between Lindanathi and Luthando, the living and the dead-as-ancestor. When he is finally circumcised, Lindanathi visits Luthando's grave: "It was a clear day and I didn't say much to him, down there. We never had to use words to discover an understanding between us" (161). However, the novel ends with an apostrophe to an addressee who is both the reader and, ultimately, Luthando:

> Bhut' Vuyo never explicitly reminds me of my promise, but I remember and live through it each day. My promise, what I told them then, is the same thing I'll tell you now. My name, which my parents got from a girl, is Lindanathi. It means wait with us, and that's what I plan on doing. So in the end, I guess this is to you, Luthando. This is your older brother, Lindanathi, and I'm ready to react for us. (161)

The exploitation of the Benvenistian pronoun "I'll tell *you*" as a shifting signifier connects reader and Luthando as co-constituents of the being of Lindanathi through the reading of his narrative. It is also a conversation between the living and the dead, one that enables a vision of unboundedness in this life through conversations with a form of subjectivity yet to come, one that is singularly *not* a fantasy, either in the form of an unattainable future or in that of an idealized past. Thus, Lindanathi is "waiting with" his community, not for an impossible good life, but for whatever may come next for any of them. It is not what-should-come-next that concerns him, but the *being-with* the community for whatever it realizes will have happened, and therefore whatever comes next. This immunity to an addiction to the good life is not masochistic; after all, Lindanathi greets the news that the government is going to provide treatment to one hundred thousand HIV-positive citizens with skepticism, as mentioned above, but not complete belief or despair: "Who knew, I thought. It was enough to believe them for *now*" (157; emphasis added). Similarly, Lindanathi makes it clear that the arrested virus in his blood does not make him a modern miracle: "I was still reactive, just slow to develop the [AIDS] syndrome. I have a large number of antibodies, for reasons the two of us couldn't fathom" (157).

I conclude by pointing out that Lindanathi chooses to live with people whose values he shares, by moving from the city to Bhut' Vuyo's shipping container in Dunoon. That is to say, I am not claiming that his form of effluent resilience is shared by his compatriots or even his friends in Cape Town. He has every opportunity to join the growing Black middle class, but he not only feels uncomfortable and unfulfilled with this "lifestyle"; he also later becomes aware that the form of labor he takes when he takes on writing for the Net is not sustainable. When he works for the Laboratory, he explains that he lives in a flat in Mowbray opposite a bar, whereas,

> my colleagues, on the other hand, had families. They had satellite TV and good skin that could flush red with gratitude. They were well adjusted and easy to admire.
> Even those who came from places redolent with defeat—District Six, Bo Kaap or Bonteheuwel—were happy with what they had. I often felt scrutinized by them, and inadequate when we cornered each other in the hallways. Nothing was lost in the silence of our elevator rides. I'd greet my co-workers with a grin, feeling myself expand with the need to rush after them and apologize for something I hadn't done. (120)

Lindanathi, then, does not belong to the speakable good life, in which health is defined as the ability to work, and in which "the African" is supposed to be grateful to the philanthropic French boss of the Technikon's lab, who sees his scientific mission as helping "Africans," whom he defines as perpetually in health and economic crises. Indeed, even when Lindanathi gets work writing for the internet on hygiene issues, he is let go in a restructuring, in which he conceives of the boom–bust cycles of capitalism: their effect on the workers such as himself, and the very unsustainability of the system, both structurally and in terms of his desire to endure the ups and downs, which does not exist:

> The directors led us in a brief discussion of the slow growth of the digital economy, explaining why redundancies were inevitable across the board. . . . In the dark I began to feel as if this crisis meeting, in which my colleagues and I had sat mostly silent, was something that had taken place before. This sense of déjà vu would only fade months later, when I saw that the restructure they'd had in mind included disposing of half the human staff, and that the

content was now collected from different sources across the Net. I realized then that the feeling I'd had at the meeting had arisen from the fact that, even as we sat in the ninth-floor boardroom that day, we'd formed part of a historical moment that had receded.

Much like light travelling from the sun, although it had seemed immediate, it had taken time to reach us: the event itself had taken place. We were already obsolete. (122)

Lindanathi, it turns out, has a keen sense of the quotidian crises of capitalism that Haigh documents and about which Berlant theorizes. He never does work in the corporate economy again. He works briefly, part-time, at a movie rental store, purveyors of entertainment used, in Berlant's terms, to interrupt the brutal discipline of self-development in moments of lateral agency; and he ends up working at the informal shantytown spaza shop, distributing free condoms with the approval of the owner and other goods as he sees fit or feels the urge to do so. The designation of obsoleteness within the colonialist-capitalist economy opens a door in which he seeks to identify reactions within himself that render him noninstrumental, and therefore not able to be made obsolete. To "wait with" the living and the dead—the work *he sets himself*—avoids assessment of him by self or others in terms of a colonialist-capitalist vision of success; it also creates opportunities for creative persistence within the field of quotidian weariness detailed by Berlant. Yet it appears to be not a temporary escape from accumulation and self-fashioning, as she describes lateral agency, but an entry into an ethics of nonaccumulation and a co-constituted fashioning between self and other, one that encompasses both the living and the dead.

Haigh points to this realm of contact between the living and the dead in the momentary, farcical desire of the dying Wesley Peacock for Shelby and in the "hindsight" he experiences after death of his egocentrism as that which prevented him having children. The instantiation of the colonialist-capitalist world as the real is interrupted both by the impropriety of Wes's posthumous reflections and by Lindanathi's living beyond the imprint of capitalist consumer desire. Indeed, the figure of the capitalist as madman or trickster reverses capitalism's apparent but not exclusive normalization in *Heat and Light*. The dead Wes haunts the text of *Heat and Light*, but never receives affirmation from those in the bubble. On the other hand, Luthando, the inspiration for his brother's "waiting for" whatever comes next, including his own death, has an entire novel dedicated to him at its conclusion: "So in the end, I guess this is to you, Luthando. This is your older brother, Lindanathi, and I'm ready to react for us" (161). Should the novel's readers be included in this apostrophe, in the first-person-singular pronoun, then the instantiation of effluent community through Lindanathi's promise to "wait with us" and react outside of the bubble is effected in the aesthetics of the novel itself, which in this context, becomes an effluent artifact. I shall return to the novel as effluent artifact in the final chapter. For now, however, I want to turn to what the body, as it bears a metonymical relation to capitalism, tells us in sexual assault. How does awareness of settler-colonial capitalism enable a reading of rape as an extractive industry? And where can we locate effluent methodology in such a reading?

4

Trauma "Exceptionalism" and Sexual Assault in Global Contexts

Methodologies and Epistemologies of the Effluent

Wilson Harris defines "vision" as "capacity to resense or rediscover a scale of community." His epigraph from his "Author's Note" to his 1973 *The Whole Armour and the Secret Ladder* reads as follows:

> That scale, I would think, needs to relate itself afresh to the "monsters" which have been constellated in the cradle of a civilization—projected outwards from the nursery or cradle thus promoting a polarization, the threat of ceaseless conflict and the necessity for a self-defensive apparatus against the world out there.
> In some degree, therefore, we need to retrieve or bring these monsters back into ourselves as native to the psyche, native to a quest for unity through contrasting elements, through the ceaseless tasks of the imagination to digest and liberate contrasting spaces rather than succumb to implacable polarizations. Such retrieval is vision. (8)

I cite Harris because his notion of "vision" relates directly to my proposition of an effluent methodology for reenvisioning sexual assault, its possible prevention, and the healing we might undertake in its wake. This methodology requires linking, on the one hand, how colonial capitalism requires the polarities Harris outlines to function and, on the other (and further), how these polarities function most specifically in the sphere of sexual assault. One way of reading Harris—a willful misreading—is to think that he is describing a liberal, "civilizing" mission of search and rescue of the native entirely consonant with colonization. However, Harris, a Guyanese author, can be read productively alongside Sylvia Wynter, in that Harris sees the monsters he names as having been born at the same time as "civilization." That is to say, just as the Wynter's "genre of man" instantiates the (white) Anthropocene and its attached liberal human-rights discourse, Harris points out that "civilization" requires its barbarian others to demonstrate its superiority within the settler-colonial context. With this reading in mind, one could say that the community Harris wants his readers to resense is an effluent community: one that does not depend on the construction of others as enemies for its foundation; one that does not depend on the papering over of the appropriation of native land and exploitative labor practices such as slavery for its justification.

I look at sexual assault as an extractive industry that finds its *metier* in colonial capitalism because, as demonstrated in the previous chapter, the dual moves of land appropriation and enslavement on which it is founded treat the body as metonym of, or part of, such extractive practices. The Pennsylvania-based poet Julia Kasdorf, while describing fracking practices to me, once pointed out that they were "like" a rape of the earth. She was picking up the very practice of sexual assault as one that falls within the context of acquisition through appropriation of land from Indigenous peoples and slave labor as the foundational "principles" of colonial capitalism. In her 2013 *Therapeutic Nations,* Dian Million makes this point in relation to Canada's radically contradictory move to acknowledge the colonial history of the Indian Act and the residential school experiences while maintaining the disempowerment of Aboriginal women in the colonial culture of sexual exploitation: "It is actually gender violence that marks the evisceration of Indigenous nations" (7). The contradiction is both radical and profound: "An Indigenous gendered concept of polity," Million states bluntly, "contradicts any Western liberal governing principle still vested in a white male heteronormative subject" (7). We are left with a key question, then: How does putting sexual assault in the colonialist-capitalist sphere change our understanding and prevention of it and make the structural violence of white male heteronormative power evident both within and outside of Indigenous communities? Asking this question is not to minimize Indigenous gender-based violence (GBV) experiences (a subject that is a key focus of chapter 5), but rather takes into account Million's concept of the structural violence of the heteronormative male subject embedded in the state's positionings of sexual "trauma" and its related characterizations of perpetrator, victim, and hero-intervenors.

The liberal recognition of victims involves the notion that the victim-survivors of sexual assault have somehow to be "rescued," following colonial modes of civilization, from victimhood and stigma, and that perpetrators need to be both vilified and punished, as if they were always already perpetrators, ontologically and essentially, before their first assault. The first move of the liberal search-and-rescue mission of survivors out of their stigma actually requires them to instantiate themselves as both victims of the violence and victims of stigma in the first place. In this way, the dynamics of recognition of victimization in order to "bring" the assaulted one back into the liberal fold parallels the structural violence Alexander Weheliye identifies in those who conceive of slaves as if they lived their entire lives under the sign of abjection. Tellingly, this dynamic of recognizing victims through their instantiation of themselves as underprivileged others echoes Lauren Berlant's work on distant suffering, as we shall see. The second move, that of vilifying perpetrators as always having been barbarians, with acts of sexual assault merely the manifestation of that fundamental propensity, means that perpetrators of all kinds are always seen as such, making any rhetoric of the attempt to bring them back into the fold, to "rehabilitate" them, as ambivalent as Homi Bhabha's colonial discourse of mimicry, which highlights how the Western-educated citizen of color is almost white "but not quite." That is to say, the perpetrator is assumed to be the "barbarian" who can never be rehabilitated out of that condition, which gives the lie to sexual assault perpetrator rehabilitation rhetoric under colonialist-capitalist governance. Like the victims who must instantiate themselves as victims, the perpetrators must elocute to their predation. If they do not, they are not *not* taking responsibility; if they do, this public "confession" becomes proof of their essentially predatory nature. Of course, who gets acquitted of sexual assault and who does not is a deeply classed and racialized process to begin with.

Seeing sexual assault in the context of the structural violence of settler colonialism is an act of effluent methodology. It involves relinquishing long-held investments in individualized models of interpersonal violence and perpetrator-victim-hero formations of sexual assault, where the hero is seen as the one who looks to intervene in the process, to prevent the assault. The reader/viewer in this effluent reconfiguration is a spectator who is a potential perpetrator and/or potential victim. They are not simply a detached observer, who potentially "intervenes" from the perspective of vilifying the perpetrator or pitying the victim-survivor. Such relinquishing means demolishing those notions of what are seen to constitute safe/bubble spaces from which to watch the spectacle of sexual violence. This makes the space to pose embodied knowledges of both "victims" and "perpetrators" as key alternatives, *effluent epistemologies* from which we can derive practices of prevention and healing. In this context, the *methodology of the effluent* requires a practice of "bearing witness," in Kelly Oliver's terms (2001), rather than recognizing violence in the outworn tropes of victim–perpetrator and savior–saved dyads that actually depend on centering the spectator/reader rather than "perpetrator" and "victim" survivors. Tellingly, the hero is never the victim-survivor, possibly because the "hero" in contemporary American popular discourse is deeply male-engendered, with few exceptions. Further, the spectator/therapist is often positioned as complicit in gender-based violence as an extractive industry through the rewards of the voyeurism of spectatorship in a "rescue" economy, both affective and economic.

I begin by demonstrating how an effluent methodology has at its core an affirmation of values extrinsic to settler-colonial capitalism. Specifically, I demonstrate how traditional trauma theory structures value in discussions of the sexual assault of women and children within colonialist-capitalist terms. This structuring, I argue, is symptomatic of a traumatic reading of harm that actually acts as a strategy of containment in how we read sexual assault. It limits the kinds of victims we recognize and simultaneously restricts the scope of the issue through its rendering of sexual assault, and especially rape, as exceptional, creating its own bubble. Further, it overlooks and overwrites the subjectivities, and often the rights, of those who have been sexually assaulted, as well as the persistence they exemplify in the face of their attacks. This persistence does not conform to normate heroism, which is exemplified in the veiled subject position of cultural self, the figure outlined by the array of deviant others whose marked bodies shore up the normate's boundaries. The term "normate" usefully designates the social figure through which people can represent themselves as definitive human beings (Thomson 2017, 8).

Here we see the link between the normate and the genre of man, to which the colonialist-capitalist understanding of sexual assault conforms: spectators/intervenors in sexual assault are seen as normate; victim-survivors are not. Spectators and intervenors undermine the idea that (their) recognition of perpetration and victimization within the tropes of liberal governance is in and of itself an intervention. I argue here that the genres of such recognition, which lie within the bounds of liberal governance, are culturally complicit in revictimizing the victim-survivors and consigning perpetrators to perpetual demonization. The effluent epistemology capable of critiquing this normate concept of sexual assault both haunts the concept's formation and exceeds it, as we shall see.

I speak of sexual assault, rather than rape exclusively. I do not agree with the focus placed on rape as separate from behaviors associated with sexual assault that are not technically rape. My argument is also informed by cultures that do not see the onset of sexual intimacy as marked by penetration.[1] My approach draws on my earlier field research and published work (Jolly 2010) on the context of sexual violence against women and children in South Africa, a postcolony with high rates of HIV infection. This discussion is informed by that work, but is also situated within, and responds to, the increasing current concern over the high rates of rape on university campuses in the United States. This juxtaposition enables me to undercut stereotypes of "privileged" viewers/spectators: spectators of suffering that occurs in communities with lower socioeconomic status than that of the spectators, communities with less political agency and "grievability" in the eyes of a Butlerian state than those spectators. The privilege stems, in part, from the assumption that such spectators are not, and cannot in the future be, victim-survivors, a (false) assumption of many citizens of "developed" countries in their views of rape in the Global South. In this respect, too, the marked division between spectacular rape and normalized forms of sexual coercion that sustains the myth of relative invulnerability reveals itself to be harmful.

I draw on my current position within a university, Penn State, that is struggling to deal with a very public set of issues concerning childhood sexual predation, and simultaneously, like many institutions across the United States, seeking to meet its obligations to student rape victim-survivors under Title IX requirements that address sexual violence against female students as an aspect of gender equity in tertiary education. In 2011, Gerry Sandusky, assistant coach of the Penn State Nittany Lions football team, was tried by a grand jury for sexual abuse of young boys and found guilty on June 22, 2012, of forty-three counts of pederasty. In 1977, Sandusky had set up a charity called The Second Mile to serve underprivileged and at-risk youth. He gained access to his victims through the charity. Penn State is involved because it was on Penn State grounds that the charity held some of its activities, and because some Penn State officials have been found guilty of neglecting Penn State community members' attempts to inform them that Sandusky had been observed in unusual sites, such as in the shower with an underage youth. The university has paid several millions in restitution to the victim-survivors and $60 million in fines to the National Collegiate Athletic Association.

There has been much written about what kinds of sexual assault victims we recognize, and what kinds we don't.[2] I rehearse these issues here but focus specifically on the *rhetorical* structures of the conditions of our recognition of sexually violent practices. The rhetorical framework manifest in these structures disables certain kinds of victimization from being seen, where such victimization is seen as implicitly normate—and therefore not victimization, in a strange tautology—while simultaneously highlighting others' instances of sexual assault because those assaults are seen to violate predetermined norms. Instances that register as "exceptional" include, for example, male-on-male and juvenile rape, which are combined in the Sandusky case. I identify the mechanics of the representation of rape victimization in the United States by its dependence on the rescue trope, which is a cultural marker of an ongoing colonial imaginary. I call for a specifically effluent intervention in the reproduction of the logic of spectacular perpetrator–victim dyads as a requirement for the contextualization of sexual assault as a preventable and treatable aspect of intersectional, structural violence. The perpetrator–victim dyads that populate public discourse on sexual assault oversimplify the issue by decontextualizing intersecting systems of oppression, domination, and discrimination. They thus strategically overlook the fact that perpetrators, victims, and spectators, complicit or otherwise, are enmeshed in intersecting webs of power that express racism, homophobia, transphobia, religious bigotry, ableism/normateness, classism, and sexism as described by Kimberle Crenshaw's feminist theory of intersectionality (1991; see also Carastathis 2014).

This absence of genres in settler-colonial cultures for describing intersectional identity in the representation of perpetrators and victims occludes what John Galtung, the founder of peace studies, terms "structural violence." He defines structural violence as the violence that results in harm and limits the realization of persons' capacities but is not attributable to a single individual or nameable authority (1969, 170–71; cited in Vorobej 2008, 84). Galtung here defines "positive peace" as the absence of structural violence. When we think of violence, especially of sexual coercion, we most often think of physical violence and seek its source in the identification and often demonization of potential perpetrators. Galtung does not seek to ignore the fact that structural violence is inherently comingled with interpersonal interactions; he just insists on placing those interactions within the structurally violent context caused by what Crenshaw identifies as the intersecting network of oppressive norms. However, I differ from Galtung in his insistence that structural violence is inherently invisible. I prefer to exploit the ideas of one of Galtung's eagle-eyed discussants and exponents, Yves Winter, who argues that structural violence is not invisible per se, but has become so familiar to us that we cannot identify its operations (2012).

The genres of perpetration and victimization attendant on our customary understandings of rape as preeminently an act of interpersonal violence between victim and perpetrator are part of the framing of rape that makes its contextual structural violence—of income inequities related to colonialist-capitalist values and practices, of heteronormativity, of racism, of settler politics, of ageism and ableism—recede, not because they are inherently invisible, but because their visibility is so much part of our normate operating context, or what Pierre Bourdieu calls our *habitus*,[3] that to notice structural violence is rather like recognizing the sky as an element in our daily apprehension of outdoor physical perspectives. Rendering this normate visibility of structural violence visible for its capacity for damage, rather than allowing its quotidian facticity to go unremarked, is necessary. This requires a conscious acknowledgment and disavowal of the genres of perpetration and victimization that deeply personalize sexual assault interactions, and in so doing, actually create stereotypes of the intersubjective violence of the assault, thereby adding to the negative implications of such intersubjective violence with structural violence's heft.

The previous chapter, in its reading of *The Reactive*, highlights the danger of responsibility taking the form of paternalistic care, whether through the instrumentalism of white liberalism or the settler state, or a combination thereof. There is yet a further link between settler colonialism and the structural violence of Galtung that Joan Cock's 2012 critique of his work highlights. In her article, she points out that Galtung's concentration on processes for peacemaking between contesting parties may evade a hugely problematic phenomenon: the fact that treaties, such as those between settlers and Aboriginals, can themselves be key elements of structural violence. They operate within liberal forms of governance structures, and rhetorically offer friendship, supposedly equal commercial exchange, and land management "agreements." However, the neoliberal concept of the self that precedes them, and on which they depend, is itself a form of structural violence, in that, as Cock argues, it makes settler-state democracy coterminous with its own foundational violence. Using the Indian Treaty System as a case in point, she observes that "nothing in the most democratic idea of a 'people' prohibits it from obliterating a reality... incompatible with its [the Treaty System's] ethos and aspirations" (2012, 227). Normate humanism and the genre of the human depend upon the exact same neoliberal concept of the self.

Specifically, then, how is vulnerability constructed in settler-colonialist and capitalist democracies in ways that determine the structural violence that is rendered an acceptable part of our *habitus*? If commodity exchange within capitalism cannot take place without including or excluding sex in its ambit (a fact that we see in forms as various as advertising and human trafficking), what does this mean for the construction of both perpetrators and victims within colonialist-capitalist registers of value? Is it appropriate to read the high rates of suicide, substance abuse, sexual assault, and exploitation in Aboriginal communities in Canada, Australia, and the United States, especially in youth, as the consequence of negative interpersonal dynamics, or indeed in isolation from one another, and in isolation from the structural violence attendant on contexts of cultural genocide, in which Aboriginal indigeneity and Black self-determination may be realities obliterated by the incompatibility with the ethics and the aspirations of the settler-colonialist capitalist democracy?[4] How do we read vulnerability to both perpetration and victimization in contexts of cultural despair? I mean the term "cultural despair" to include the criterion of low socioeconomic status and to exceed it. I am talking about communities that have had their culture "obliterated," to use Cock's term, by a "reality" incompatible with its ethos (settler capitalism) and "aspirations" (full sovereignty, including title rights over former Aboriginal lands). What if we were to use effluent epistemologies to read settler-colonialist privilege as *a source of cultural despair to the colonizer-settlers* (albeit a vastly different kind of despair from that of colonized communities), rather than the "good life" colonial capitalism promises?

The refusal of Alexis Wright (whose work I read closely in the next chapter) and a myriad other Indigenous artists and leaders to see the Aboriginal as disadvantaged *only* in relation to settler-capitalist cultures[5] leads me to ask, thinking analogously: what would an approach to sexual violence prevention, treatment, and aftercare look like in a context in which women and children are not forever implicitly and exclusively conceived of as vulnerable? This is not to say that there are not whole communities that are disproportionately vulnerable to sexual violence. These include Aboriginal communities, those involved in transactional sex of all kinds, trafficked women and children, women and children in conflict and postconflict contexts, and refugees, to name but a few.[6] If, as Weheliye has pointed out, slaves do not live the entirety of their enslavement as embodied abjection, surely we can see that victim-survivors have not just subjectivity but also accompanying agency? Further, what if those assumed to be "protected" from sexual assault by their "race," socioeconomic status, and (assumed) spatial invulnerability are in fact rendered vulnerable by such assumptions of privilege? What if the bubble is actually a dangerous place?

The prevalence of sexual violence blinds societies to recognizing it as an effect of structural, rather than simply interpersonal, violence. This encourages spectators to view women and children as inherently vulnerable physically, owing to their "reduced" physical strength in relation to men. What gets lost in this approach is that women and children are *rendered* vulnerable only when they are put in positions of vulnerability through patriarchal sexism, just as Aboriginal communities are rendered vulnerable when "protected" by settler capitalism in the name of democracy. Potential perpetrators are also rendered vulnerable to perpetration under such conditions. The West's initial difficulty in grasping the fact that child soldiers are perpetrators and victims at one and the same time speaks to the addiction to an apartheid-like separation of the two categories (Redress 2006).

What makes women and children "vulnerable" is not any property inherent to the physicality of women and children, then, but the behaviors of potential and actual perpetrators in societies that register their horror at rape yet fail to address the structural drivers of sexual assault, such as massive gaps in socioeconomic status, the drivers of conflict, and the conception of women and children as property, as part and parcel of land there to be acquired, with the accompanying overwriting of dispossession that applies: in this case, dispossession of the victim's subjective and embodied integrity. What also gets lost is the fact that perpetrators can be and often have been themselves groomed in that behavior during their childhood. This is not to take responsibility away from such perpetrators, or to suggest the inevitability of their behavior. It is, instead, to acknowledge the need to look at intergenerational patterns of perpetration and victimization in ways that do not simplemindedly pose a drama of villains and victims cut off from history, isolated in an hypostasized, vicariously thrilling, and spectacularized moment in time.[7] The attractions of this genre are that the reader/spectator is set up as one who "saves," or at the very least can then see another "character" (perhaps the state, as in the case of the Northern Territory Intervention, discussed in the next chapter) going in to "save" the vulnerable woman or child, or even better, Aboriginal woman or child, who always needs saving ("child" but not "male" being the category ripe for saving, despite the possible coincidence of the two in the subjectivity of the victim). Hence the entry of heroism under the sign of the savior into the spectacular drama of perpetration and victimization through which we read sexual assault.

This paternalistic desire to save becomes evident when we see the massive concern over child victim-survivors when compared to adult female victim-survivors, suggesting that the rape of children is somehow worse on a comparative scale of harm than that of an adult woman. This has become particularly apparent to me working from the institutional context of Penn State University, which in 2012, as I noted above, experienced the Sandusky affair, the exhaustive legal and related details of which I shall not rehearse here. I am, however, interested in the surprising (to me, at least) conceptual divorce that we as a university community tend as a whole to have between, on the one hand, the issue of the sexual abuse of children that has so affected our community and, on the other, the considerable efforts we are making to address the problem of the rape of female students on and around the campus.

There seems to be a concern that to try to think through these two events together, which share a venue and a kind of perpetration (sexual abuse), is to confuse them as being one and the same event, to commit a category mistake (and, in my view, a categorical one), and further, would force into the light an implicit anxiety that to speak of them in relation to one another is to somehow contaminate "regular" heterosexual, adult rape (!) with the stigma of both same-sex assault and sexual victimization of children. I question some assumptions underlying this lack of the desire to think through these events in relation to one another. The first is the irrelevance of the supposed sexual orientation of the perpetrator to the estimation of harm.

The idea that male-on-male sexual assault is somehow worse than male-on-female sexual assault appears to me to draw from two assumptions that I reject: one is an implicit, long-standing, and deeply disturbing association between same-sex desire and pederasty, a profoundly absurd association in view of the incidence and prevalence of heterosexual pederasty; and secondly, an implicit notion that the rape of children is somehow a worse judgment on the community than the rape of adult women, an approach that establishes a hierarchy of harm: raping a child is worse rather than a *different* outcome of a same behavior, in that both perpetrations manifest sexual assault.

The Spectacle of Child-Rape Exceptionalism

The approach of child-rape-victim exceptionality rests on refusing to think through some admittedly challenging issues; but this refusal resurrects a set of false values in its attempt to isolate the issue of sexual violence in disaggregated spheres. First, infants and children who are raped are seen as having been violated, whereas the sexual assault without penetration of children should be seen as equally pernicious in its own way. This leads us to one dubious outcome of constructing rape as "more extreme" than other forms of sexual assault: the physical evidence of penetration enables voyeurism in a distinctive way, in that it offers an ongoing or remaining sign of the act on the body of the victim. Further, an associated implication of child-rape exceptionalism is that adult women are somehow more able to prevent themselves from being raped than children in all cases, a preconception that is often false, based as it is on the notion that women are always more able to escape men's aggression than are children. This assumes personal physical strength of the victim to be not only a relevant issue, but *the* determining factor in sexual assault. Further, the notion that the harm done to an infant or child is somehow "worse" than that done to an adult woman risks normalizing the rape of woman as somehow more acceptable than the rape of children, and implies that adult recovery from rape is less traumatic. Clinically, as the South African experience demonstrates, the harms cannot and should not be ranked in terms of harm: their outcomes are both harmful, but very different.

For example, an infant on a colostomy bag caused by the rupture of their genitalia and digestive tracts through rape has a physical harm that is enormous; yet such infants can recover social interaction and faith in community far more readily than children attacked as they head toward puberty and upward.[8] Further, infants, children, adolescents, and women require radically different forms of therapy after assault, as those working with children in communities of high prevalence of sexual assault have pointed out. For example, children often need and wish to talk about the experience with community members, whereas their parents and other elders, in an attempt both to contain stigma and protect the children from stigmatization, often attempt to censor this much-needed discussion. Children can show extraordinary resilience here: while their elders attempt, albeit for good reasons to do with prevention of stigmatization of the child and family, to prevent childhood sexual abuse from entering the speakable, quotidian, discourse of the community, children both want and need to take a different tack, especially when the aggressor has in the past threatened the child with violence if they speak of the sexual aggression. Once the threat of retaliation is removed, the speaking child can do much to heal both self and community. I should emphasize, here, however, that I am not underwriting "the speaking cure" as a panacea for all trauma victim-survivors. I am suggesting that we take a lesson from child-rape-survivor resilience in the model of speaking sexual assault back into the fabric of quotidian life, rather than spectacularizing it through censorship and rendering what I call its effluent quality secret. The idea is not to "traumatize" a public, but to make childhood sexual assault speakable for the benefit of the community, including the child survivor.

Reading Gender-Based Violence as an Environment

I am not suggesting that the kind of out-of-the-box reading I propose here is an easy switch in gears. For those of us who have worked in the applied contexts of massive and enduring trauma, the attractions of reading trauma as a series of singular, catastrophic events are multiple. I speak here from decades of experience of working with victim-survivors of state-sponsored torture in the aftermath of South Africa's transition to democracy, and with victim-survivors of gender-based coercion and abuse in South Africa during the height of the HIV pandemic, of which the area of KwaZulu-Natal (KZN) in which I worked was an epicenter. The experience of the HIV context was instructive. There was 33 percent prevalence, according to prenatal testing statistics, at the time. Working alongside the medical professionals, traditional healers, spiritual groups of various sorts, and welfare systems, both government-funded and NGO, we learned that HIV positivity was not an event, but an environment. People were dying more quickly than their families could afford to bury them properly, the hospital morgues and incinerators were overwhelmed, and surgery took place in a context of double-gloving and repeated postexposure prophylaxis that left visiting surgeons from the northern hemisphere feeling scared, underskilled, and clumsy. No one ever died of AIDS, as the stigma was so great that officials producing death certificates would kindly choose (or be bribed into) writing "TB" as the cause of death; and in any event, one doesn't die of AIDS, but of opportunistic infections.

HIV and fear of AIDS were the fabric in which we lived and worked within a quotidian set of challenges that refused to frame themselves nicely around the genres of individual diagnoses, discrete tragedies, and personal fear. Rather, the experience was of communal exhaustion, communal fear, unspoken but perennial stigma, wild swings between despair as to the usefulness of our work and absolute belief in its essential contribution, and unholy delight in dark humor that formed an element of communal resilience. This is certainly not to claim that individuals were not isolated by virtue of positive HIV diagnosis, or that communal experience trumps despair, or humor triumphs over HIV. Not at all. It is merely to say that HIV was an environment in which events happened; it was not a discrete event in and of itself. And this is still the case today, although the environment has been changed by the introduction of maternal-child prophylaxis, more broadly available HAART treatment, and a change (although not an eradication) in the profiles of stigma in rural communities.

One night, on field research, I had a deep and heated argument with two of my colleagues, one a Canadian South Africanist of decades' standing with a partner but no children, the other a South African–born Zulu mother of three children. I myself have a partner, but no children. I was making an argument I later put into print, about the fact that I believed the rape of a woman versus an infant is neither better nor worse morally, just different in its clinical outcomes and victim-survivor service needs. We were struggling with the fact that South Africa, a country with one of the highest sexual violence statistics in the world, was expressing horror and disgust at the "events" that came to light in 2002–2003 of multiple infant rapes, usually of infants neglected momentarily or for stretches of time by mothers and grandmothers who were themselves impoverished, lacking social supports, and sometimes substance abusers. The rapists were most frequently gangs of deeply marginalized (homeless, unemployed, substance-abusing) men and boys.

My sense of offense at this response of horror and shock to the "event" of infant rape had to do with the fact that the infant rapes could be considered exceptional only if one were to ignore the prolonged and sustained history of violence against *women* in South Africa. Indeed, the infant rapes are part of a continuum of violence that is intergenerational and has deep roots in the entanglements of colonial, neocolonial, and postcolonial racist and sexist violence, including the particular forms of familial breakdown coerced into being by the racist forms of industrialization under the European colonial governments and the apartheid regime, not to mention the systems of slavery and indentured labor that undergirded that development.

My Canadian-born South African colleague steadfastly maintained that infant rape would always in some sense be "worse" than the rape of adult women, whereas my South African–born colleague-mother referred to her own motherhood and then stated that "you're right, Rose; but we can't go there with you yet in our minds. It's too hard to bear." This argument was vehement and fueled by the stresses of working in an environment structured by both endemic HIV and gender-based violence and coercion, just as much as racism. I see both my colleagues' responses as attempts, in a sense, to prevent the spread of gender-based trauma out of what is perceived to be the exceptional horror of infant rape and into the broader spectrum of gender-based violence, including sexual assault of females and males, children and adults. This response may also reflect an investment in framing our research subject (GBV) more in terms of a series of "events" rather than a structural challenge, in order for us to make GBV prevention and the provision of services for its treatment "manageable" in order for us to employ a bubble-type strategy of containment.

Indeed, this notion of illness as event rather than environment more broadly construed is a limitation public health itself is confronting, as fifth-wave public health theory attests. Fifth-wave public-health theory, discussed in further detail in the following chapter, argues that the major challenges for public health in contemporary times are themselves symptoms of modern ways of life, and as such, are compound challenges that do not offer the cause-and-effect simplicity of, say, John Snow removing the handle of a water pump to curtail the outbreak of cholera in 1854 Soho in London. We did come to conceptualize the project's understanding of GBV as a continuum, in which, for example, the societal acceptability of verbal abuse, which is often regarded as less offensive and therefore more acceptable than physical abuse, cannot be separated from "events" of physical GBV, including but not limited to rape, as the physical cannot be extracted from the context constituted by the systemic oppression of infants, girls, women, boys, and men perceived for whatever reason to be challenging masculinist, heterosexist authority.

Being in one of the first teams in rural KZN to work on gender-based violence in HIV settings, with that conjunction as a driving factor of the research, made me realize how valuable this experience of HIV as environment, not event, was. In 2003, when we began the GBV work in earnest, the largest concern was an event-based understanding of the rape of women and children as *the* traumatic event. This was supported by the series of child- and infant-rape scandals that were hitting the newspapers in South Africa at the time, as well as the heritage of the tendency of the Truth and Reconciliation Commission (TRC) to view a girl or woman's rape as the "foundational trauma" of her testimony. As with HIV, GBV is similarly not simply a series of events, but an environment in which we work. Female victim-survivors understand this in their rejection of the formation of rape as the foundational trauma of womanhood, indicating their essential vulnerability and gendered identity. This attitude meant that men whose torture had taken the form of object and other kinds of rape who testified at the TRC never bore witness to being rape victim-survivors: they would say they were tortured, but not raped, further consolidating the erroneous notion that a woman's inherent physiology makes her a potential or actual rape victim but men cannot be raped, an obviously false aspect of a disturbing heteronormative configuration of rape. The man cannot be raped, because then he becomes feminized.

Subsequent work on the TRC—that of Fiona Ross, Antjie Krog, and my own among others—has since registered and objected to the expectation of how women were to talk about their sexual assault (Krog 1998; Ross 2002; Jolly 2010). These expectations involved requiring a woman to speak of her sexual assault as if it were a nonsystemically generated event, but rather "personal," and as if there were no life after rape for the woman and as if rape is still currently (at the time of testimony) the woman's greatest challenge (as opposed to the crises of food security for her children or education for them). Feminist critiques of these expectations have since gone some way to dislodge the assumption of "the rape" as *the* foundational trauma of the lives of girls and women who suffer a series of traumatic events in their lives, and who did/do not always see their rape (or rapes) as emblematic in the way in which the deeply gendered views of the

TRC trained that community to hear as foundational traumatic events in testimony.

Such is the power generated by the generic expectations of readers and listeners: that it can willfully reshape testimony within the testifier's repeated, explicit, and accessible protestations to the contrary. The momentum to override victim-survivors' self-expressed needs is symptomatic of paternalistic approaches that assume victim-survivors, whether adult or child, lose their brains along with their entire sense of self at the moment of victimization. Further, the dependence on how those other than the victim-survivors construe the traumatic "event" also plays into hierarchies of victims: why are certain rapes worthy of reporting in the newspapers and others merely attributable to the generalized violence of the poor, the racialized, the Aboriginal-ized, and the lower classes? One response would be that the need to confine trauma within the bounds of discrete events is symptomatic of imaginations that either cannot or refuse to construe systemic oppression as traumatic because it does not conform to the "event" model, as such construal would indeed be "trauma out of bounds," as Stef Craps has suggested (2013). Trauma out of bounds, which is what I am advocating here, sees violence, including sexual assault, within the context of structural violence, the context of the structural violence under my lens being settler-colonial capitalism. Our focus, then, is not a foundational traumatic event, but an environment in and of itself.

The "Value" of Foundational Events in Narrative and Diagnostic Trauma Theory

The history of the development of trauma theory can be seen as a history of repeated substitutions of the investments of viewers, readers, and audiences, often professionals attached to these activities, such as critics, doctors, therapists, psychoanalysts, archivists, for those of the traumatized subject(s) whose interests such professionals and other empathetic persons assume they are supporting, or even advancing, in their descriptions of traumatic events. While others have pointed out the problems with the constitution of trauma as an event, rather than a series of "quasi-events" with no beginning or end in sight, we owe it to ourselves, as humanist scholars with aspirations to humanitarianism, to take into account the ways in which the genre of trauma as singular, overwhelming event emerged in the academy as an interest of a group of humanist scholars at the same time that the humanities themselves were being broadly recognized to be "in crisis," owing to their inability to conform readily to instrumentalist assumptions about what should constitute the proper "job" of tertiary education.

Trauma theory coming out of humanities departments in the 1980s and 1990s linked traumatic event to narrative in ways that invoked a particularly strict sequence of tense in narrative that I contend has arguably more to do with the power of modernist/postmodernist paradigms in Western humanities departments, dependent upon a core set of culturally specific and obviously culturally apprehended "crises," such as agnosticism/atheism and the Holocaust, than it has to do with identifying a transhistorical and/or transglobal set of narrative forms that can be confidently associated with either the diagnosis of trauma, on the one hand, or its "working through," on the other. This has to do with a substitution of a particular configuration of the relations between trauma and narrative in Western academies for the task of imagining trauma otherwise, elsewhere, and in other times. The tendency of trauma theory to short-circuit its own ethical potential through invocation of the exigency of the trauma in question, or what I think of as an addiction to the genre of trauma as a singular, overwhelming event, is a repeated pattern in the hiccupped history of its development.

One of these hiccups has to do with the fact that an addiction to the generic understanding of trauma as a singular event demands exemplary singular events, the choice of which immediately bears witness to the colonial imaginary of the Western academy: the identification of such exemplary events is deeply logo-centric, the Holocaust or 9/11 being cases in point. In this dependence on a "founding trauma," the trauma is offered as a founding experience for an individual or a generation, but it emerges as the founding trauma, or at most a set of founding traumas, depended on by the theory itself, and well within the investments of the North American academy in terms of its archetypal referents. That is to say, what is determined as an archetypal referent says more about those determining it to be archetypal than it does about what a global economy of trauma might look like, were the dominance of Western catastrophe to be somehow neutralized. For example, while Dominick LaCapra acknowledges the centrality of the Holocaust throughout his work, and acknowledges that the focus on the Holocaust could indeed mask unpalatable traumas closer to home, such as slavery (and, we might propose, "rape" or sexual assault culture), he nevertheless asserts that "slavery, like the Holocaust, nonetheless presents, for a people, problems of severe traumatization, a divided heritage, the question of a founding trauma, the forging of identities in the present, and so forth" (2014, 174). Craps comments on this insistence on a foundational trauma and its dubious claims to comprehensiveness via analogy: "Slavery, apartheid, and the atomic bombing of Hiroshima and Nagasaki are occasionally mentioned alongside the Holocaust—for example, as instances of 'founding trauma'" (2013, 81), but "in general these other histories play a very limited role in [LaCapra's] book" (10).

Here I argue that the remedy is not one of simple supplementation—add non-Western traumatic events and stir—but a critical investigation of how the traumatic event came to be defined as such within the confines of Western academic and medical collaborations over the definition of event-based/foundational trauma. The selection of sexual assault as a test case makes the limitations of traditional trauma theory even more visible than the easier-to-render analogies of slavery, apartheid, and the atomic bomb, largely because the personalization of sexual assault within the genre of the "foundational trauma" highlights its isolation from considerations of structural, intersectional violence. This insistence on a foundational traumatic event, rather than a *sequence* of events, can have negative consequences in the treatment of childhood-trauma survivors, where children who experience one traumatic event demonstrate far more resilience than those who experience repeated trauma, even when ensuing trauma is not necessarily (repeated) sexual assault.[9]

I once cosupervised a PhD student who insistently wanted to research the violence endured by women in rural KZN within the framework of interpersonal violence (IPV). The wish was particularly to research whether women were being beaten by their intimate partners particularly when they disclosed to those partners that they were HIV positive. Despite my advice to the contrary, the student decided to run a set of interviews on this question. I fully acknowledge that the investment as a PhD student in public health was informed by the fact that the IPV model was (and in some places, remains) the dominant model for addressing partner violence. But the questionnaire responses provided little by way of connection between "I am HIV-positive" and "I am being abused," to the extent that this approach had to be abandoned. This was because women do not necessarily know why they are being beaten, especially in a context in which what is called IPV occurs both prior to and after events that we might think of as key beginning and ending points, or founding traumas, such as an HIV diagnosis; the women themselves experience the abuse as duration, not as an event with a beginning and end. Further, one cannot assume that perpetrators "know" why they are beating their partners. *There is, in this sense, no founding traumatic event.* The contextual factors in this case are the dispossession of Black, rural men under British colonial and apartheid regimes, the continuance of that dispossession after apartheid, and the colonial teaching, entrenched in Black communities by the long *durée* of various forms of colonization, that respect is a zero-sum game (Jolly 2010).

The "founding trauma" concept is codependent with definitions of traumatic events as they are given in medical terms, most especially in the *Diagnostic and Statistical Manual of Mental Disorders*, now in its fifth edition (*DSM-5*), which has a history of moving from earlier conceptualizations of diagnoses such as post-traumatic stress disorder (PTSD) as based on a singular event that occurs as an exception to quotidian experience to a new concept of multiple-traumatic-event exposure. While the *DSM-5* has expanded the singular-event conceptualization of traumatic syndromes, the conceptualization has maintained its paradigmatic status in both diagnostic manuals and trauma theory concerned with outlining the relation of narrative to traumatic event, even where it is recognized that multiple-traumatic-event exposure can occur.[10] Once again, I suggest that this is in part the role the humanities took during the rise of trauma theory to define narrative studies in terms of the late-capitalist logic of the *usefulness* of trauma, since a narrative event or symptom, such as silence, conforms to the generic configuration of trauma as a medical event: both can be identified, recognized, and in fact "diagnosed," then treated with pharmaceuticals and/or various forms of narrative therapy.[11] Most notable in terms of influence in this regard is indeed LaCapra, whose work on the Shoah has been instrumental in contemporary constructions of how to read silences not only in fictional narratives, but in personal ones (see for example, LaCapra 2016, 2004, 1994). Further, the categorization of trauma as event-based, rather than environmentally contextualized through intersectional readings of structural violence, will never be able to see trauma within the framework of fifth-wave public-health theory, as traumatic experience is the symptom, and the environment itself the cause.

Event-based trauma analyses, then, are consonant nonintersectional "diagnoses" of rape as nonintergenerational and isolated from other events of sexual assault and abuse.[12] These diagnoses may have been overdetermined by concentration on the classifications of the sex and/or sexual orientation of both perpetrator and victim, and age of victim, as I argue happened in the Sandusky case. In the remainder of this chapter, I reflect on changes required to situate "trauma" as a valid term within actual sexual assault victim-survivors' lives. In order to register the impacts of both structural violence and intergenerational trauma, I propose we need to rethink perpetration and victimization in terms that exceed the individual, and ditch assumptions that trauma attaches only to the victim side of the perpetrator–victim dyad. That is to say, *we need to see ourselves as having been traumatized, the symptom of which is our insistence on seeing victim-survivors as having had exceptional experiences.* What's in it for us in adopting this false view is that it enables us to overlook the ubiquity of sexual violence in order to, first, render ourselves safe both from conceiving of ourselves as potential perpetrators or victims and, second, have a containment strategy that views rape as exceptional so it can continue to believe that the normal life excludes not only rape perpetration and victimization, but also gender-based coercion of all kinds.

Traumatic Histories within a Global Comparative Framework: Deconstructing Spectator/Reader Privilege

To see traumatic events as part of ongoing histories of oppression, rather than exceptional events—inconceivable, immoral ruptures in the fabric of history—is in part to expose the assumption that persons grounded in the supposedly relatively "safe" spaces of the "first" and "second" worlds have access to personal safety. It is also to encourage comprehension of complicities in both perpetration and victimhood that exceed the present moment and the category of the individual. In other words, we need to reconceive of traumatic time and space as the spatial, temporal, material, spiritual, and political reality that many inhabit, not as a singular event visited on them in a past that needs to be put in the past, narratively speaking, for the trauma to be "worked through" "successfully."

If, as Rob Nixon argues in his 2011 *Slow Violence,* what makes environmental harm so challenging to recognize is its failure to conform to the genre of the singular, spectacular, traumatic event, instead revealing itself in the scales of intergenerational (or even geological) time and in nonspectacular increments, then I am proposing we consider the slow violence of living within sexual-coercion trauma: trauma as an experience of cumulative "quasi-events," as Elizabeth Povinelli terms them, rather than *the* traumatic event, such as sexual assault, as a singular, spectacular exception. The failure of the imagination posed by the exceptional approach, I have argued above, has to do with the refusal of the privileged, or more accurately *self-assumed privileged,* observer of the trauma to see the traumatic event as exemplary of certain forms of catastrophic, unsustainable structural violence. Here, the trauma observer prefers the fetishization of victimization *without* the entanglements of radical, systemic transformation that would change the material, intergenerational conditions of the structural violence that produce traumatic duration as (intergenerationally) lived experience, and without framings of traumatic experience and resilience as *mutually inclusive* categories.

Berlant offers one of the most trenchant critiques of trauma theory focused on trauma as event. Her argument appears to be akin to Povinelli's, in that they both reject the extraordinary, singular identification of trauma described in the work of LaCapra and Cathy Caruth. What such critics see is the failure of trauma theory to account for suffering that is "ordinary, chronic, and cruddy rather than catastrophic, crisis-laden, and sublime" (Povinelli 2011, 3). Povinelli writes from her position as a companion both in social projects in the United States and in daily life with the Aboriginal inhabitants of Australia, while Berlant confines her critique, explicitly so in her 2011 *Cruel Optimism,* to the Unites States and Europe. In Berlant's case, the turn away from trauma theory is grounded in the understanding that trauma-as-singular-event entrenches a liberal sentiment based in a profoundly conservative optics of spectacularized suffering, described in her 2001 "Subject of True Feeling." Yet her work depends on an assumption that the spectators in such instances are already living, or believe themselves to be living, in a context of relative privilege and isolation from the time and space of the catastrophic events. This means that *the spectators always envision themselves as observers of atrocity, in this case sexual assault, including rape, and not as potential victims or perpetrators.*

Further, while it does not explicitly make this claim, Berlant's work (both "The Subject of True Feeling" and the subsequent *Cruel Optimism*) appears to assume that all relatively privileged citizens of the late liberal era (or those who identify themselves as such) can address the suffering of the other *only* through a politics of recognition that frames bearing witness to such suffering through the optics of sympathetic subject and traumatized "object." (Whether this is because she actually believes this to be so or because it's the only dynamic she describes, remains unclear.) Her references in this instance include issues such as child-soldiers in Africa and garment workers in India; she points out that the vast geography of such an optics of sympathetic spectacularization prevents solidarity between members of communities at home in the United States, when disparities in wealth and other resources result in what I am calling, after Povinelli's influence, the "grotty" trauma of the quotidian (2011, 3).

Berlant's compelling reading of trauma in "Subject of True Feeling" positions the spectator as politically embedded in late liberalism in a commodity culture that cannot deliver on the promise of the "good life." In her configuration, the suffering spectacle or object, which is actually the *primary* subject of the trauma in her argument, is displaced/misplaced elsewhere either spatially, temporally, or both; she is either too far away or too close to home to be recognized within an actual politics of affect grounded in communal resilience; she is either the incinerated garment worker (too far away) or the single mother, imprisoned for being too poor to pay fines (dangerously close to home in terms of pure geographical proximity, perhaps, but distanced by the barriers of an assumed middle-class decency.) What Berlant overlooks is yet another "switch and bait" move in the development of trauma theory and its responses, in that she writes as if all North American inhabitants have *only emerging genres* of how to deal with their own suffering under late liberalism.

This is an assumption that carries its own late-liberal misconceptions in the name of displacing those very misconceptions, in that many Aboriginal, postslavery, and migrant postcolonial communities have intergenerational knowledge and the genres to go with them capable of apprehending the late-liberal present not as a deepening shadow whose genres have yet to be developed for it to be understood, but instead as a belated repetition of colonial trauma proper to those who invested in the state and individual property rights in the first place. This does *not* include all North American inhabitants. Here I am thinking of Aboriginal literatures that include reproductions of administrative authorities as naive to the point of foolish, as we see in Wright's Uptowners of the next chapter, or Armand Ruffo's Catholic priest in the film *A Wendigo Story*. I am also thinking of how Wright and Ruffo's narratives not only know but also embody the fact that colonialist culture brings with it the patriarchy of entitlement through not only land ownership, but also the presumptive ownership of women's and children's bodies under the guise of patriarchal protection. I am also thinking of the conventional reading of Appalachian communities as apathetic in their apparently mystifying refusal to either "develop" or "be developed," without an understanding that their relation to their land is one of co-constituted identity over generations, which makes moving to take up work in a city or destroying the land in the service of industrialization inconceivable—they refuse neocolonial-capitalist "protection" in its destructive capacities.

When the abuse of women and children in sexual violation is mourned in many social spheres, it may *appear* as caring for those victims as persons; but it may also in fact *be* outrage at the rape of bodies presumed to be in the ownership of, and under the protection of, the patriarchal family and its mirrored structures in the state and university governance. This means that, when sexually aggressive behaviors, such as Trump's self-described "locker room talk,"[13] coincide with the identity of the president of the country, he appears in public discourse to be comparatively exempt from the outings of the sexual coercion and assault of other men of his generation. We have yet to see, then, whether the current outing of hyperpowerful men as predatory in the United States under the "#Me Too" movement actually eventuates into changed structures of business and governance that have hitherto formed pathways for accepting and managing the fallout of high-profile accusations, such as nondisclosure agreements paid for by companies and the U.S. government.

Patriarchal protectionism explains to some degree why the sexual assault of students has become such an issue in recent years, in that students are associated with the stereotypical vulnerable subject: they are young, are away from the presumed (but not necessarily actual) safe space of home, often have reasonable-to-good socioeconomic status, and are adolescent. In this respect, the Obama children were the exemplary potential victims "in need of" protection. As adolescents, university students are conceived of as that impossible subject who is both supposedly autonomous yet entrusted to the university for "safe-keeping." Trafficked women, Aboriginal women, migrant women, and those of other low-socioeconomic-status groups are far less numerous on a campus such as mine than are middle- and upper-class women whose families can afford a university education, or at least afford, or think of affording, the debt burden that follows in its wake. This makes me suspicious of the isolation of the campus rape from other spaces and places of sexual violence in North America. While I would never turn down advocacy to prevent rape anywhere, including university campuses, this does not mean that I cannot view critically the recent focus on female students. Are such students more valuable than trafficked women, in the same way that children are perceived of as more "valuable" than adult women when it comes to rape prevention? Is the exercise in "saving our female students" yet another performance of the patriarchal desire to "save" the child from becoming damaged goods, rather than to pay attention to the structural violence of patriarchy itself?

These are women who receive a double message from society and parents alike: be whatever you want to be *and* don't get pregnant; don't get raped; don't get drunk; don't become spoiled goods. Or, as one State College high-school student explained to me, "My parents tell me I can be whatever I want and go wherever I want; but they also say I mustn't go near Penn State on football weekends because I won't be safe." This contradiction takes a slightly different form in rape-prevention work on campuses: women must be careful not to get drunk or imbibe liquids laced with rape drugs such as Rohipnol, *and* if sex is forced upon them without their consent, even if they are unable to form consent, the man is responsible, *but* because the law is based on consent being formed or not formed between two people, and the inebriated cannot form consent, these cases have notoriously low prosecution and conviction rates. At stake is who is in a better position to claim the protection of citizenship.

Think, for example, of the repeated scandals of football players being released from potential prosecution for sexually assaulting women because of the commodity value they hold for their institutions. While such players may indeed be regarded as privileged in this situation, the fact remains that, even as perpetrators, their status as commodity, just as their purported victims' status as commodity, is what makes their fate a context they share with those purported victims, not a consideration of them as human beings on a perilous trajectory from adolescence to adulthood.

There is a vulnerability to perpetration, but it manifestly lies too little in the area of consequences when commodity value is at stake. We see this vulnerability play out spectacularly in cases in which gifted players from underprivileged backgrounds are suddenly thrown into the spotlight owing to their commodity value for their universities. Any youth navigating such a dramatic change in social, cultural, and material circumstances would find this challenging, let alone in an environment such as the United States. The common reluctance to discuss racial privilege, among other forms of inequity, in the name of a supposedly already-achieved nonracialism in the sports arena, as well as the fact that talking about it with affected individuals is difficult, makes such discussions exceptionally challenging, if not virtually impossible. Here the presumed remaindered or "effluent" player is rendered a full citizen supposedly through his "gift," but actually through the value of the *commodification* of that gift. What is rendered effluent here is the adolescent himself: he "falls out of" the fiction of full manhood, fully gifted, full citizenship. In this respect, the $950k paid by the University of South Florida to the purported victim of Jameis Winston can be seen as a form of fine for refusing to deal with Winston-as-effluent as opposed to Winston-as-sports-hero, winner of the Heisman and other trophies.

My point is *not* to call Winston an effluent character in terms of Judith Butler's current theories of disposability or ungrievablity. Indeed, his salary in 2017 was $615k. Instead, I aim to supplement Butler's argument by claiming that those seen as valuable through commodification, such as sports heroes, themselves become nongrievable in that their failings or losses can be registered only ever in relation to their performance *as players*, in relation to their commoditized value. That is to say, their failures are regarded as threats to, or actual loss of, their commodity value. I am not giving my key term, *effluence*, a negative connotation, but precisely the opposite: once the patronizing spectacularization of victims and the demonization of perpetrators is put in context, one can see that what remains *in excess of viewing the perpetrator or victim as a commodity* is that which *has value in and of itself,* regardless of social bias: the *remainder-as-effluent.*

Indeed, one can use Povinelli's concentrations on the *tense* of late-liberal notions of citizenship to construct a decolonial critique of some of the assumptions that frame Berlant's nevertheless astute observations about the conservative workings of sentimentality in the wake of the entrenchment of trauma-as-event as the dominant genre for managing suffering—more specifically, the suffering of "others"—in the United States in the past three decades. One can also use the debate I am staging between the work of Povinelli and Berlant to begin to frame the questions: How do we begin to envision *what is left out in framing suffering as either failing or that which is "ordinary, chronic, and cruddy"*? How do we frame effluence outside of this binary? How is sexual assault not exceptional, and how do we deal with that fact without confusing the ubiquitous with the acceptable? (Not that Povinelli makes this error, it should be noted.) In other words, how do we describe a world in which the spatiotemporal distinctions between that ordinary, chronic suffering and that which is catastrophic decrease rapidly and occasionally collapse into one another?

This "remainder," or "effluent," as I call such unspeakable collusions between catastrophic and cruddy, is important material. Its connections between the quotidian and the meaningful event are capable of giving the lie to formulations of chronological time on which the projects of eschatological Christianity, empire, nationalism, and late liberalism all subsist; and the genre of trauma-as-event lies *within* this deeply limited framing of tense. To bring it home: for the trafficked woman, the woman in an abusive relationship, the child in an abusive home, sexual assault is not normally a rape, but a continuum of abuse that includes multiple rapes and other forms of sexual assault; and she knows she may well not be valuable enough to command respect in this situation, let alone a successful chance of prosecution of her abuser. In many instances, it may be more comforting to suffer the abuse than risk society reminding her of how valueless she is by refusing to hear her voice and/or refusing her the material conditions to escape her abjected world.

The remainder, meaning the conjunction of the cruddy and catastrophic in which the actual experience of repeated trauma, including sexual trauma both from perpetrator and victim positions (which may well be exchanged through time), also suggests ways in which we can begin to address the suffering of others outside of the framework described by Berlant. That is, we can begin to conceive of bearing witness to suffering in spatiotemporal formulations that *exceed* the structure dictated by the optics of spectacularization, with its attendant substitution of the seen suffering (the raped child, for example) as object in place of the subject, the viewer as the never-have-been and never-to-be perpetrator or victim. Further, we can begin to think beyond spectacularization's attribution of the suffering of the privileged-world viewing "witness" as invariably the consequence of secondary trauma produced by the suffering of those with whom s/he is not co-incident (the rape victim of disaster in a far-flung corner of the world; the rape victim in the sociopolitical apartheid of the slum next door; the raped student; the sexually abused child). Indeed, we can begin to see the politics of spectacular witnessing as dependent on a refusal to see the viewing subjects as themselves mired in traumas properly attributable not only to the cruel optimism of late liberalism, but rather to late liberalism as a product of colonial commodification.

The politics of spectacular sympathy produces the suffering of the privileged-world viewer as secondary trauma. Secondary trauma is commonly defined as the effects of seeing a traumatic event in which one cannot intervene or cannot intervene to the benefit of the victim(s). This formulation of secondary trauma can actively disguise a form of suffering *on the part of the viewer that is primary to that viewer and related to their embeddedness in a set of values that always produces material wealth as a place of unsufferability.* The history of late liberalism not only as cruel optimism, but as product of colonial commodification, provides an alternative in terms of a historical long *durée,* or prehistory, to that which Berlant outlines.

This history and the critical genres for its telling are available in the form of the persistence of communities who live, and have always lived, outside the promise of the (eventual) good life proffered by the supposedly redemptive teleologies of colonization and its descendant, late liberalism. These redemptive technologies can be named, in view of this alternative history, as a set of ways of being in the world that are profoundly neocolonial in their material, moral, and social regimes. This is the knowledge, the epistemology, of those who already know themselves to be effluent, in the sense of being immaterial to the ruling regimes and genres of commodified settler colonialism.

Effluent Epistemology as a Basis for Sexual Assault Prevention and Healing: Body-Mapping and Forum Theater as Effluent-Enabling Interventions

With this effluent option for reenvisioning the meaning of sexual coercion and assault on the horizon, I now return to the challenge I posed earlier: the need to extend trauma theory beyond its Freudian origins in the therapist–victim-survivor dyad and the Western juridical and moral models that tend to assign trauma only to the victim side of the perpetrator–victim dyad. Michael Rothberg points out that "the categories of victim and perpetrator derive from either moral or legal discourse, but the concept of human trauma emerges from a diagnostic reality that lies beyond guilt and innocence, good and evil" (2009, 90). The problem here is twofold.

First, it would be appropriate for Rothberg to say the concept of human trauma *should* emerge from a diagnostic reality that extends beyond guilt and innocence, good and evil, rather than to claim that it *does.* That is to say, much of the energy and ethical imperative or urgency of trauma studies is invested in advocacy on the part of the victim-survivor; exploring the intergenerational condition of systemic trauma that leads to victims becoming perpetrators is a far less popular activity. Victim and victim-survivor support are far more attractive than the preventative resources that lie in the histories of perpetrators.

Second, to see traumatic events and their perpetrators as parts of ongoing histories of oppression, rather than exceptional events that erupt as inconceivable, immoral ruptures in the fabric of human history, entails a reworlding of the genres of modernism and postmodernism. A modernist rhetoric of origins that resurrects the crises of human morality in terms of secularism, industrialization, and the First and Second World Wars, is a profoundly Western set of generic concerns. It also depends on an eccentric, not to mention absurd, alliance of the integrated psyche of the individual with a mythic original wholeness fractured by the (very culturally specific) crises of Western modernism.

The refusal of the trauma of the perpetrator also rests on a transnational appeal, unfortunately not nearly so globally specific, to the socio/psychopath as the common perpetrator of traumatic harm—Harris's "monster"—rather than the perpetrator who either is a victim-survivor of systemic harm or is trained to perform that harm through professional or other modeling, or both. It is always a relief to my students when I explain to them that the specialists in the "dirty tricks" of the apartheid regime had to be trained to overcome their aversion to torturing, maiming, and killing other nonhuman animals: they started with small rodents and worked their way up through dogs and horses to violence against humans. They required training to overcome the common inhibition to wound others. While humans are not inherently moral, they are not inherently bound toward violence either. Of course, there are sociopaths who inflict traumatic harm; but professional torturers for the most part require training to overcome basic inhibitions against the deliberate maiming and killing of others.

The refusal to explore the trauma of the perpetrator has much to do with a terror of perpetratorhood trauma expressed in moral terms. Yet this terror, like the terror attached to infant rape, both masks our refusal, in lateral terms, to acknowledge communal perpetratorhood and victimization in conditions of structural violence in which we become complicit, often with little awareness of doing so, and masks our refusal, in historical terms, to identify intergenerationally with entangled histories, presents, and futures of perpetratorship and victimization. It's far easier to delimit the subjectivity of victims and perpetrators within the containment strategy of individual subjectivity. Easier by far to contain the traumatic event to a singular moment in time. However, this means limiting sexual-coercion prevention to a structural inequity in which females are always encouraged to see themselves as potential victims, whereas men are not encouraged to see themselves as potential perpetrators because they are too busy being told how to save young women from rape as a prevention strategy. Why would any young man ever be brought to see himself as a potential perpetrator within the steadfast vision of man-as-protector posed by the majority of prevention programs? Why the steadfast avoidance of "shame" in the instantiation of the perpetrator and the endurance of cultures of "shame" around victim-survivors?

In my 2010 *Cultured Violence*, I argued that there is a reason for the supposed shame experienced by sexual assault victim-survivors. I rehearse and add to that argument here. Following Butler, the rape victim-survivor is often seen to be ashamed. In the apprehension of the victim-survivor who seeks anonymity as if she had herself "done something wrong," the world of speakable discourse, following Butler, implicitly realizes this retreat from public view as a recognition of her devaluation. Yet, in feminist terms, it is seen as the ramblings of the insane attributable to the unspeakable, in that the raped subject "should not" see herself as ashamed. The lack of meaning comes from the notion that she, the victim-survivor, is in fact insane to attribute blame to herself within feminist terms. However, in this quintessential moment of misrecognition by a public entrenched in the structural violence that devalues victims, the survivor loses the witness to her harm that Oliver argues is so crucial to the affirmation of those who bear witness to their own violation: "Our experience is meaningful for us, only if we can imagine that it is meaningful to others. Creating or finding meaning for oneself is possible only through the internalization of meaning for others" (2001, 83).

Giorgio Agamben, drawing heavily upon the writings of Primo Levi and others in relation to survivors of the death camps, argues in his 1998 *Homo Sacer* that the shame experienced by the survivors is not that of "survivor guilt," because it has nothing to do with the culpable states of either guilt or innocence. Instead, this shame derives from "being assigned to something [let us say, using Oliver's vocabulary, a subject position] from which we cannot in any way distance ourselves" (105). Here shame is specifically *not* an assertion of responsibility on the part of victim-survivor for her violation; it is instead her registering of the *impossibility of her distancing her-*

self from the subject position to which she has been consigned by a publicly constituted visibility that sees her exclusively as (the raped) woman. She sees herself being seen as that which is not coincident with her sense of herself.

This moment is characterized by the double movement in which, simultaneously, the subject, by instantiating herself as a subject within what Butler calls the domain of the speakable, is at that very moment witness to her own desubjectification:

> Here the "I" is thus overcome by its own passivity, its ownmost sensibility; yet this expropriation and desubjectification is also an extreme and irreducible presence of the "I" to itself. It is as if our consciousness collapsed and, seeking to flee in all directions, were simultaneously summoned by an irrefutable order to be present at its own defacement, at the expropriation of what is most its own. In shame the subject thus has no other content than its own desubjectification; it becomes witness to its own disorder, its own oblivion as a subject. This double movement, which is both subjectification and desubjectification, is shame. (Agamben 1998, 105–6)

The framework constructed through a theoretical triangulation of Butler, Oliver, and Agamben allows us to read such shame as the victim-survivor's recognition of her own irrelevance to the social order in which she finds herself. This irrelevance is thrown in her face when her violation cannot be registered because she is, at best, a quasi-subject, whose violation is therefore a quasi-violation—itself, tellingly, an impossibility. As we have seen, the victim-survivor's awareness of her impropriety as a subject in the order in which she finds herself is registered by her, in narrative form, in the tropes of shame in terms of the public view of her. The tropes that appear when she reflects on her own position of being an impossible subject are those of insanity.

The healing task then becomes the engagement of the effluent remainder of this process: the sense of self of the victim that lies *between* the social sense, the structurally violent forms of shame and abjection, and the crushing subjective perception of one's abject status as constructed by those forms. This is a tiny space, and in my experience, it requires trust and great skill on the part of the survivor and their allies to grow that space. It also requires cohort-building among victim-survivors who have themselves borne witness to their own desubjectification, overcoming the trauma of that desubjectification through sharing the experience of it with others who, in Oliver's terms, affirm the subject's experience. In this context, I find two of the activities most proven to succeed in this arena are forum theater and body-mapping, as both provide space for mutual affirmation and exploration of the roles and effects of perpetrators and stigmatizers consonant with structural violence on the collective beings of survivors. The opening of this space is accomplished through the persistence of the effluent, which in this specific context I define as an embodied epistemology of co-constituted subjectivity that exceeds the double moment of subjectification and desubjectification of Agamben, which is does by creating alternative modes of affirmation: modes of affirmation that are not defined by the coincidence of the speakable and the insane in the construction of the violated subject as, simultaneously, not supposed to be feeling shame ("it's not your fault you were raped") and absolutely supposed to be feeling shame ("there is something about you that makes you improper, something you did that enabled you to be violated, despite the order of our lives, so we approve when you exhibit the appropriate shame in our presence. It relieves us").

Forum theater, pioneered by Augusto Boal in the 1970s, is used to enable youth to develop a body language (which ultimately moves to include spoken language) to communicate what survivors see as the key issues in their communities. Following Butler's research on the speakable as the terrain of the empowered/unstigmatized, it follows that new gestures, new languages, or very old languages not usually recognized within the sphere of the normate are needed for survivors to express their fears and desires outside the realm of the speakable, which brings with it the gaze of judgment and censorship that restricts activities of self-expression before they can even be thought. Groups are encouraged to use their bodies to interact with one another in the first instance *without* spoken language, to enable novel languages of movement and attitude to be borne and/or practiced. They then develop scenarios that express their thoughts, fears, needs, hopes, and dreams using each other's bodies to formulate the gestures of a story. Eventually the story is developed into a basic scenario in which any participant can "roll back" the action to produce a different outcome. In this sense, forum theater provides an arena of communal rehearsal of scenarios feared and dreamed, enabling survivors to envision themselves differently: not simply as reactors to an oppressive set of institutionalized judgments, but as literally authors of their own stories, for which they seek reflection and support from their survivor cohort as commenters, intervenors, and enablers. The movement from survivors' perceptions of themselves as actual or potential instruments of exploitation can be navigated instead through self-perceptions of decision-making ability, skills-building, self-esteem, and empathy needed for positive outcomes in the face of serious forms of structural violence.

Body-mapping takes place in workshops of eight or thereabouts. It originated and was used in mapping the progress of early highly-active-antiretroviral-therapy (HAART) patients who are HIV-positive in South Africa, where the body-maps did bear witness to scenes of GBV, despite the explicit focus on HAART (Solomon 2008), and has been piloted in an initiative to support survivors who are writers and poets in Cape Town and Buenos Aires. Each workshop participant works on a life-size outline of their body, supported by trained facilitators; or the facilitator draws the outline. The participants then fill in their body-maps in relation to a series of carefully queued questions about personal histories, vulnerabilities, and areas of resource and resilience. No previous art training is required, although the body-maps can turn out to be striking. Body-mapping is a very intimate space, and the appropriate supports, such as special ethics for highly vulnerable populations, the potential for triggers, and other potential supports needed arising from body-mapping are planned for in advance. The process produces cohort-building among stigmatized groups and a strong sense of how survivors see their bodies and how they see themselves being seen by others and raises consciousness of these self- and social lenses.

With the permission of the creators, the body-maps and some portions of the forum theater—usually advanced segments of the performance workshop—may then be used to facilitate group and community discussion at the level of structural determinants of vulnerability, impossibility, support, and possibility. That is to say, they can be presented in facilitated workshops in which potential and as-yet-unidentified actual perpetrators of gender-based violence are offered the opportunity to bear witness to the effects of its structural and interpersonal harms. These activities have more hope of success than normate behavior-change interventions, many of which are based on a model of "Don't do this" because it is illegal or morally wrong or will be bad for you, as opposed to an approach that explores the realm of what can happen if *one* (the third-person singular generic, not the potentially accusatory second-person *you*) does engage the spectrum of gender-based violence in the full range, from implicit verbal threat to explicit sexual assault. (Here I am also careful to explain that the range does not imply a range of less to more damaging behaviors, as harmfulness depends on more factors that involve both rhetorical and physical violence in all their combinations thereof, and is context-specific to each case.)

I would additionally propose that these activities are also highly valuable to undertake with groups in which unidentified perpetrators, victim-survivors, and potential perpetrators and victim-survivors, as well as those who may have occupied both positions at different times, are likely to be present. I once was involved in a forum theater workshop with youth at high risk of perpetration and victimization in gender-based violence in rural KZN. I remember two scenarios vividly. One occurred when we asked the youth to give us "body pictures" of the troubles they saw in their community. They set up what was obviously a shebeen (informal pub) scene where, in a valley away from the scene, one young man viciously raped another, to the extent that his body movements made us aware that he had either raped or been raped or had witnessed the episode at close hand. However, the point is that he was able to demonstrate his knowledge of the violence *outside* of the economies of judgment and censorship that terminate youth's ability to explore what they witness in crucial forms of playacting.

On another occasion, I was aware that one young man was teased by the others as having some sort of alternative gender identity, although I was unable to put my finger on what exactly this was; it could have been anything on a range from LBGTQA to having been a recognized victim-survivor of GBV (or both; I couldn't say). My isiZulu is far too basic to catch nuances of this sort, and the extralinguistic cues the others were exchanging among themselves and with him were not within my capacity to "read." He consistently refused to volunteer himself as a role player in the forum theater process, until toward the end of the day, when he inserted his body in a montage, or "still life," made up of the other participants in various stances. At the last call for those present to "play," I inserted my body next to his, and with great caution, extended my hand toward his in such a way that if he rejected it, no one could easily see the gesture. I was, after all, a white workshop facilitator, and he was a young Black man for whom the post-apartheid stakes of our relative positions could not be more loaded. Nevertheless, to my surprise, he grabbed my hand and held on to it so hard that his fingers left marks on my skin, at the joints of my fingers. To this day I do not know whether this was a pull of support or something else entirely, but I do know it was the only responsive gesture the participant made in the course of a two-day workshop that I saw in the context of the workshop activities: and whatever it may have meant, an emotion was intensely expressed.

I remember being melancholically sad at one team member's response when I recommended that our team should interview perpetrators of GBV from the local prison. They said in outraged tones that they had no intention of dedicating time to "converting sex offenders" (presumably to the ways of gender equity). I had no intention of such a goal. It was a research team and I was looking to see how patterns of victimization and perpetration repeat themselves in specific sublocales of the district in which we worked. This story tells me once again how quickly we jump to judgment before we understand anything about the forms of structural violence that produce GBV perpetration. This means that we rarely, if ever, arrive at deep, differentiated, and subtle understandings of how to change the parameters of structures in which GBV is, as I have argued before, cultured rather than contested. Imagine what Jameis Winston could tell us about the conditions of elite-university-sports-team perpetration were he ever offered the opportunity to do so without further incriminating himself in the network of big-player-makes-it-good-then-shows-his-real-self, his supposed innate violent and racialized masculinity (with his status as "sports hero" recovered through the re-covering of that "real self" in his recruitment by the Tampa Bay Buccaneers despite the accusations of sexual assault and abuse from his university days). Within the making-invisible of structural violence, the knowledge of the effluent—that which could enable us to address the violence of the structure—is lost to us. The making-invisible of structural violence appears as a form of resilience against harm; but like so many outworn structures of self-preservation, it has not only lost its applicability, but in fact also renders us all quintessentially vulnerable, "privileged" and exploited alike, albeit differentially. As Million's work suggests, naming structural violence without sufficiently describing its mechanisms in a specific context is yet another way of obscuring its operations in that context. Effluent methodology and epistemology offer settler cultures different frameworks for conceptualizing, and therefore developing preventative strategies for, sexual assault in settler- and postsettler-colony contexts. In my final chapter, I present a reading of Wright's magnum opus, *Carpen-*

taria, that attempts to deploy the aspects of effluent visions I have touched on here and in the previous chapters: mourning the dead in an intergenerational, animistic milieu in a way that is indeed generative (chapter 1); understanding what illness and its antecedents look like from an effluent perspective in the postcolony (chapter 2); naming the ethic failures of extractive industries in relation to the earth and the body (chapter 3); and sexual assault in the postcolony, as well as the rhetoric that papers over failures to apprehend the effluent in it (chapter 4). Let's see what the entire architecture of the effluent vision looks like in a practical application of it to that most elusive of forms, a radically decolonial manifestation of the novel.

5

Effluent Capacity and the Human Right-Making Artifact

Alexis Wright's Carpentaria *as Geobiography*

> *For many indigenous peoples, their nonhuman others may not be understood in even critical Western frameworks as living.*
>
> —Kim TallBear, "Theorizing Queer Inhumanisms: An Indigenous Reflection on Working beyond the Human/Not Human"

Alexis Wright's award-winning novel *Carpentaria* locates practices of Aboriginal life in the space of harm reduction as a necessary response to colonialist-capitalist regimes of governance. To reiterate, I use the term "colonialist-capitalist" in the light of work on capitalism and territorialism such as Giovanni Arrighi's 1994 *The Long Twentieth Century* (esp. 159–214) to foreground the fact that, as noted in the introduction, to quote Elizabeth Povinelli, "whether of an American, British or Chinese shape, all imperial undergarments of a capitalist expansion have a similar cut, namely, accumulation by dispossession" (2011, 18; citing David Harvey). Or, put another way, capitalism requires (often unacknowledged) subventions from forms of colonialism and neocolonialism entailing land grabs and forms of unfair labor practices, such as slavery and indentured labor. "Harm reduction" is a term taken from public health approaches to substance abuse, where it's assumed that an addictive pattern will repeat itself, prompting the question of how the supporters of the patient can make sure as little damage as possible happens during an inevitable next abuse. Here I use the term to describe a set of practices Wright delineates in the novel as actions taken by Aboriginal communities to persist in the face of Western cultures of governance that deny Aboriginal ways of living in their colonialist-capitalist assumptions. Colonialist governance depends on normative rights regimes, as we have seen in the concurrence of Sylvia Wynter's "genre of man," the normate of the liberal human, and the normative genre of the human in the 1948 United Nations *Declaration on Human Rights* (UNDHR) and its related documents.

I use "anthropocentric" rather than "normative" in the rest of this chapter to underwrite the exclusion of Indigenous life from the UNDHR and its conventions. While it is true that the United Nations drew up its *Declaration on the Rights of Indigenous Peoples* (UNDRIP) in 2007, the declaration is neither a convention nor a treaty, and therefore has to be adopted into a country's legislation to become binding. Primarily at issue is clause 19:

> States shall consult and cooperate in good faith with the indigenous peoples concerned through their own representative institutions in order to obtain their free, prior and informed consent before adopting and implementing legislative or administrative measures that may affect them.

Prime Minister Stephen Harper of Canada accepted the statement only as "aspirational," since what is known as the "FRIC" ("free, prior, and informed consent") provision stands in contradiction to the Constitution of Canada, particularly with regard to economic development. Australia, New Zealand, and the United States took the same stance as Canada. For all practical intents and purposes, then, the generic "human" of the UNDHR, to the extent that it has been adopted by its signatories, bumps UNDRIP provisions, rendering Indigenous peoples as secondary to settler-colonial subjects. Further, the human-rights approach denies the extra-Cartesian basis of Aboriginal being as co-constitutive between human, nonhuman animals, and what we call the environment. The approach depends on what Kelly Oliver has identified in her 2001 *Witnessing* as a "politics of recognition": only those who do not have human rights may need to seek them; when they do seek them, provision of those rights depends on the terms set by the granting authority. Those seeking rights are necessarily interpolated as supplicants within the normative human-rights framework, since that framework was itself not constructed with the free, prior, and informed consent of Aboriginal peoples.

Carpentaria posits a human right-making framework as the outcome of what Povinelli terms "Aboriginal labour." Right-making activity in *Carpentaria* depicts human right-making as a practice that exceeds the colonialist-capitalist imaginary, not least because, while in no way antihuman, the practice does not center the human. *Carpentaria* does not anchor human rights to the nation-state, either. Rather, it frames all beings, including non-carbon forms such as rocks, as constituted through their intersubjectivity. If the human animal is to survive, other nonhuman animals and the resources the earth provides must also survive in human right-making's intersubjective construction of being, an intersubjectivity akin to that proposed by Es'kia Mphahlele's African humanism. *Carpentaria* itself comprises a right-making artifact of the same kind, for which it implicitly argues. It thus posits a new relation between literature and human rights: one in which right-making intersubjectivities and the literary forms that manifest them constitute quintessential decolonial critiques of normative human-rights narratives.

I begin my argument with the notorious episode of Australia's Northern Territory National Emergency Response (NTER), in which a state-sanctioned set of rights-bearing institutions decided to intervene to "ensure" the "rights" of Aboriginal communities, especially children. This contextualizes Wright's novel in an Australia that has made an apology for the incarceration of children in residential schools but simultaneously has undertaken an intervention that contravenes the UNDHR in stripping Aboriginal citizens of their rights as Australian citizens. Here the rights-seeking subject is concocted in the national imaginary (as is so often the case): the Aboriginal child who is forever the victim of (Aboriginal) sexual assault. The paternalistic dynamic of the intervention speaks directly to the politics of liberal recognition so carefully critiqued by Oliver and demonstrates the willingness of the settler-colonial state to intervene "on behalf" of Aboriginal children framed as victims of their communities' predatory sexual behavior. Here the children become the stereotypical victims described in the previous chapter, and the state the patriarchal hero that intervenes in the acts perpetrated against them, even though the state itself is an institution of structural violence in that "the abject heart of colonialism and capitalism, and their practice of capitalism, is gendered violence.... Gendered violence is perpetuated by individuals and polities at times when ... there is a threat to the power still invested in a racialized white male universalized subject" (Million 2013, 177).[1]

The Northern Territory Emergency Intervention

The NTER has been justified by the supposed failings of Aboriginal communities to protect children in their communities from harm, most particularly sexual assault. As is now widely known, the NTER followed the publication of the *Little Children Are Sacred* report (commonly known as LCASR), commissioned by the Northern Territory Government, on the protection of Aboriginal children from abuse (Anderson and Wild 2007). Authors Patricia Anderson and Rex Wild made several recommendations in the report framed firmly within an understanding of the intergenerational violence colonialism generates, a sense that solutions would have to be well funded by sustainable resources provided by the national and territorial governments, and the idea that collaboration between Aboriginal and governing bodies from the ground up, rather than a top-down approach, would be essential to solving the problems of child sexual abuse in the Northern Territory.

When the Howard government did act, their intervention was far from the careful recommendations of the report. The NTER effectively suspended Aboriginal self-determination principles through the NTER Acts; the Families, Community Services and Indigenous Affairs and Other Legislation Amendment; the Social Security and Other Legislation Amendment; and the Appropriation Acts 1 and 2 of the NTER (2007) in its suspension of the Australian Racial Discrimination Act (RDA) of 1975. In essence, the government stripped Aboriginal communities of human rights. It removed the permit system for access to Aboriginal land, abolished government-funded Community Development Employment Projects (CDEP), subjected Aboriginal children to being taught in a language they don't speak for the first four hours at school, quarantined 50 percent of welfare payments, expected Aboriginal people to lease property to the government in return for basic services, acquired Aboriginal land by compulsion, and subjected Aboriginal children to mandatory health checks without consulting their parents.

The NTER Acts of 2007 were followed by the Stronger Futures bills of 2011 and 2012 (the Stronger Futures in the Northern Territory Bill of 2011, the Stronger Futures in the Northern Territory [Consequential and Transitional Provisions] Bill 2011, the Social Security Legislation Amendment Bill of 2011, and the Stronger Futures in the Northern Territory Act 2012), which, while repealing some of the egregious "special measures" provisions of the 2007 NTER Acts, still lacked a "notwithstanding" clause requested by the Australian Human Rights Commission (AHRC) to ensure that, in cases of ambiguity between the Stronger Futures bills of 2011 and the RDA, the latter shall prevail, as shall Australia's compliance with the International Convention on the Elimination of All Forms of Racial Discrimination (ICERD). However, while the Stronger Futures Act is "intended to operate, and to be construed, consistently with the Racial Discrimination Act," it nevertheless holds that the "tackling alcohol," "land reform," and "food security" measures are all "special measures" within the context of the 1975 RDA (Australian Human Rights Commission 2011, 26). The AHRC argues that deeming these measures to be "special" supposedly demarcates them as nondiscriminatory, a position with which the AHRC does not agree. Against the Stronger Futures approach, the AHRC argues that these measures "purport to have a protective purpose for some Indigenous people, or some members of Indigenous communities, but operate by restricting the rights of some or all of the members of those groups or communities" (7).

The NTER and its subsequent iteration, Stronger Futures, can be (and has been) seen as the consequence of the "failure" of Aboriginal communities in and on what is often assumed to be the equal, or equalizable, playing field of colonial capitalism. This is apparent specifically when we understand that the Stronger Futures Act seeks privatization in the area of land occupation and the granting of special licenses for the distribution of food and alcohol in areas affected by the legislation. The NTER has been assessed in this context as the *failure* of contemporary Australian governance structures to support environments in which Aboriginal communities can thrive, as the government deploys paternalistic and assimilationist strategies of government intervention, and is accordingly criticized by not only Anderson and Wild but also numerous scholars such as Peter Billings (2009) and Alissa Macoun (2011). The NTER manifests the Australian government's demands for Aboriginal communities to conform to "normalized" governance strategies (Altman and Russel 2012; Morphy and Morphy 2013). The government response to the publication of LCASR ignored every recommendation in the report to construct local solutions in tandem with Aboriginal communities. It did so because, as a settler-colonial government, it is built on a structure that presupposes "accumulation by dispossession" (Harvey 2011, 67). The figure of the sexually abused child was nothing more than a convenient stalking horse by which to continue such dispossession.

Reframing Human Rights and Literature: From Rights-Bearing to Right-Making

When many of us are taught how to think of human rights, we tend to think of them in their idealized forms alongside Gross Human Rights Violations, with the human as a singular subject at the core of the project.[2] But how can we reimagine the right to access health, the right to free association, and the right to self-determination in an extra-anthropocentrically conceived world in ways that are *not* simplistically configured according to the impossible gap between, on the one hand, the UNDHR and its associated proclamations and, on the other, how those rights are regularly violated on the ground? What are our *actual* resources for building both ideas and practices of extra-anthropocentric human rights reiteratively? What happens if we move away from the ideals of human rights and toward *making* extra-anthropocentric human rights? This is crucial from the perspective of the unsustainability of anthropocentric human rights, not because we cannot afford for everyone to achieve the good life under colonial capitalism (although, as I shall explore later, this is indeed true), but because as a species we need to negotiate a sense of rights in relation to nonspecist and ecological sets of values precisely for the human itself to be sustainable.

Joseph Slaughter (2007, 4) proposes that the human-rights conventions of the UNDHR and its related legislative conventions share with the novel—and in particular, the bildungsroman—a subject. In both cases, this subject is proposed as commonsensical and available to all; but the constitution of the subject requires the work of literary and cultural forms to make sense of human-rights norms, which are simultaneously a fait accompli and a work in progress. The genre of the human is not an aspect of the essential human, then, but is *fictional*, having a character that itself can change. The very construction of character, its resistance and malleability, and its vibration, as it were, in the face of seismic changes in our sociocultural fabric, has to be described for us to understand an argument such as the one Slaughter makes. The subject of narrative discourse, be it explicitly fictional or not fictional, is always, in its radical sense, fictional.

I use this radical feature of the subject to contest Marianne Hirsch, among others, that the bildungsroman continues to serve as "the most salient genre for the literature of social outsiders, primarily women or minority groups" (Hirsch as cited in Slaughter 2007, 27). As I noted in the Introduction, while the bildungsroman continues to serve as the most apprehensible genre to those inured to reading within Wynter's genre of the human, it is not necessarily the most salient genre for "minorities" of that vast variety of subjects rendered marginal to liberal human discourse in the first instance. Why is the most salient genre for such "minorities" inevitably the one in which "we" (a liberal, globalized/metropolitan reading public) understand "them" (the "losers" in the current global order) best?

Carpentaria reframes the argument on the relations between literature and human rights. One example of the exploitation of Aboriginal labor for colonial capitalism purposes is represented by one of the Aboriginal protagonist's, Normal Phantom's son, Kevin, who is intellectually brilliant but of necessity takes a job at the mine and is a victim of an accident on his first day that leaves him severely disabled (and easy "prey" for the bullying of racist white boys who, dressed in Klan-like hoods, drag him behind their car and leave him for dead). Less direct than this are the unflinching representations of three abandoned, glue-sniffing Aboriginal kids who are imprisoned instead of having their actual needs addressed. The white community is too concerned with other issues at the time, such as the egg-laying capacities of their hens (a comical yet poignant reminder of the dependence of some forms of production on nonmechanized and therefore strangely vulnerable life: instrumentalization does not guarantee predictable production outcomes where carbon life forms are at stake). While these children are not direct victims of the Gurfurrit mine as Kevin is, their behavior can be seen as an entirely understandable response to the prospects for Aboriginal youth that Kevin embodies. To put it bluntly, if one is to be consumed by colonial capitalism anyway, one option of a brutally limited range is to choose one's own method of self-consumption and make it pleasurable, as in an escape, should such an escape be possible.

Within the humanities, focus on colonization as a singular traumatic event, or at least as the most overwhelming factor of quotidian life in Indigenous communities, tends to overlook questions of intergenerational Indigenous knowledge, questions of environmental sustainability, and functions of resilience. Such postcolonialism-as-trauma employs the narrow, medical model of (putatively diagnostic) narrative, in which a discrete symptom or set of symptoms is identified with insufficient reference to the complex physical, social, and nonmaterial environment in which it appears.[3] If I were to ally myself with the kind of medical model that needs to encapsulate trauma as a singular event that we diagnose and then treat,

I would fail to read the self-harming practices of the Aboriginal youth within the intergenerational, historical framework I posed in chapter 2. I might read them, instead, by applying a liberal individualist approach to the "flawed character" of Aboriginal youth. This would, however, be a reading complicit with the notion that Aboriginal youth live in an environment in which their choices are not constrained or "disabled" (Andersson 2006). Concomitantly, such a reading cuts off the possibility of interpreting Aboriginal youth's self-harm as potentially resistant to a colonialist-capitalist system that will consume them anyway in the not-so-long run, as Kevin's case evidences, and *on its own terms* at that, meaning according to an agenda in which Aboriginal youth have no substantive say.

Readings of character-as-symptom cannot in fact adopt a decolonial politics, precisely because they enable the systemic or structural violence of colonial capitalism through their inability to render that very violence as itself the ailment. They offer us the pathological Aboriginal in its stead. Even where the postcolonial character conforms to the model of the bildungsroman to access human rights, there is a sacrifice, in that the structural violence of colonialism, which brings normative human rights and human-rights violations in its wake, can be obfuscated. Tsitsi Dangarembga's *Nervous Conditions* is a case in point here: for every Tambudzai, there is a Nyasha who cannot tolerate the conjunction between colonialism and patriarchy that "saves" Tambudzai from obscurity. Nyasha experiences Anorexia and psychosis, to use the pathological terms of character, rather than the effluent ones of colonialist-capitalist harm. Indeed, Wright's refusal to parade her (non)characters in the traditional camouflage of characters as we are apt to recognize them—within the genre of the human, or what Slaughter identifies as "personality development" (2007, 4)—can be read as a further prompt to read subjectivity in *Carpentaria* outside those tropes.

Harm Reduction as Bizarre Persistence: Colonial Capitalism and Fifth-Wave Public-Health Theory

I have argued above that healthy character corresponds to rights-bearing subjects, whereas those assumed to be rights-seeking subjects (in this case, Aboriginal children) are posed as victims of a pathological "Aboriginality" within the colonialist-capitalist structure of the NTER. In this section, I advocate fifth-wave public-health theory as a model for understanding the damage of these normative readings of rights-bearing and rights-seeking subjects. I resist reading the Northern Territory Aboriginal communities as inherently pathological, the (mis)interpretation of the LCASR that justified the intervention in the first place.[4] While a narrow understanding of the medical concept of resilience might read suicide rates, substance abuse, and other forms of self-harming behavior as signs of an inherent or pathological failure of Aboriginal communities, a clearer understanding of what substance abuse and related self-harming practices in communities such as those around the Gulf of Carpentaria might *mean* in relation to resilience is proposed by contemporary public-health theory, to which I turn briefly as a resource for how to open up our possibilities of reading the three imprisoned youth of *Carpentaria* otherwise.

Some contemporary public-health analyses reject framing health challenges faced by current globalized communities as events that can be addressed from within extant conceptions of public health. These challenges are best understood, public-health advocates argue, not as diagnoses so much as symptoms of the unsustainable ways of living promoted by late-capitalist political, material, and sociocultural practices of being in the world. These ways of being and the (failed) promises attached to them form a "fifth wave" of public-health challenges, in which public-health interventions per se have diminishing returns in an environment in which late capitalism and the ways of being in the world it habituates *are themselves the ailment*, not the secondary "infections" they produce: overwhelming poverty, substance abuse, malnutrition and overnutrition (leading to obesity), unemployment, and a host of related "conditions" (Hanlon et al. 2011).

In this context, the boys' substance abuse is not a symptom of their illness, but a consequence of colonial capitalism as an ailment in and of itself. Conversely, reading the boys' substance abuse as inherently pathological, according to the genre of character and its mutually sustaining narrow medical model, actually enables overlooking the construction and conditions of labor "offered" by the mine. Further, the boys' substance abuse can be read as a complex element of resistance to colonial capitalism. If their choice is between, on one side, working under the conditions Kevin endures and, on the other, preempting that eventuality through a self-destruction that offers pleasure in the moment and is, on top of that, in direct contravention of the white Uptowners' values, then their option to harm their bodies in advance of those bodies being turned into fodder for the mine makes sense: a sense analogous to that of the slave who murders her own child, or babies born into slavery, to protect those children from slavery. Both acts pose as unlivable the utilization of the Aboriginal/Black body as, materially, the subvention capitalism demands from colonized/enslaved bodies.

If white settler readers shrink from this reading, we need to consider that we may actually be shrinking from the impossibility Wright confronts, that of healthy Aboriginal living under colonial capitalism's terms. Arguments to the contrary may express what we (want to) see: the empowerment of the boys to choose otherwise, to choose to preserve their bodies. Assumption of this possibility, this camouflage, disables the question of the boys' abducted sovereignty through their instrumentalization and exploitation within the colonialist-capitalist economy Wright details. It is worth remembering, in this regard, that Wright's first foray into nonfiction work, her 1997 *Grog War*, was on the struggle of community elders to restrict the selling of alcohol in the remote community of Tennant Creek, against the wishes of licensees and the broader community. It is also worth noting that Wright has spoken and written incessantly against the NTER, as its encroachment on the sovereignty of the Indigenous people of the Northern Territory is fundamentally unacceptable. She has stated repeatedly that the challenges facing the Northern Territory cannot be solved effectively without appropriate self-governance.[5] In this light, Australian colonialist-capitalist governance represents the condition of late-capitalist governance that is itself the ailment, and the addiction and self-harm epidemics faced by the Northern Territory communities are symptoms of that ailment: this is fifth-wave public-health theory at work in conjunction with anti-colonialist-capitalist analysis.

One could view my argument about the self-harm of the glue-sniffing boys of *Carpentaria* as a kind of obverse of Berlant's "cruel optimism," a "relation that exists when something you desire is actually an obstacle to your flourishing.... These kinds of optimistic relation are not inherently cruel. They only become cruel when the object that draws your attachment actively impedes the aim that brought you to it initially" (2011, 1). Berlant is describing a present after the world wars and the affective disorders in it, which stem from the inability of the West to deliver on the promise of the good life that is the unquestioned yet generally unattainable goal of liberal-capitalist societies. In an obverse reading of Berlant, we could imagine a kind of enjoyable pessimism in desiring an obstacle to one's flourishing, a kind of masochistic registration of the fact that one is never going to be able to "have" the good life in terms of one's current position within the liberal-capitalist economy. However, I would argue that this obverse simply does not work in relation to *Carpentaria*'s Aboriginal community, the "*down*towners," since they do not appear to either desire or be persuaded by the good life in the first place, as we shall see in the case of old man Joseph Midnight, who comes to reject his company-built house as poison, preferring to live in a shack nearby.

I propose that the Aboriginal youth of *Carpentaria*, unlike either Berlant's cruel optimist or their obverse, the masochistic pessimist, understand the system itself (liberal capitalism) not only as one within which the good life is unobtainable by/for them, but as one in which *others'* belief in the fantasy of the good life *for themselves* entails the instrumentalization of *Aboriginal bodies* in high-risk manual labor, a fact of which they arguably have an *embodied, intergenerational knowledge* through the experience of colonialism. In this context, self-harming behaviors can once again be seen as neither cruel optimism nor pleasurable pessimism, but as the bizarre persistence produced by those who intimate at the embodied level that the self-destruction of their bodies is a preemptive act of agency in a system that will otherwise use those bodies in processes of slow death to keep others' putative belief in the good life going.

Staging Geobiographical Value: *Carpentaria*'s "Timescape"

The extra-anthropocentric values posed by *Carpentaria* assist us in articulating a framework for extra-anthropocentric human rights, which include but exceed the rights of "the human." They do so by assuming that human rights need to be a set of practices, not a possession; and they include centrally, not peripherally, those whose value systems are not consonant with property rights and other forms of entitlement through possession. Within some Aboriginal artifacts there reside value systems that prove to be resources capable of actualizing extra-anthropocentric, human rights, while they defamiliarize capitalist normalization.

Carpentaria deals in extramaterialist meanings, aesthetics, and value systems, intergenerational knowledges, and timeframes that do not distinguish between "Life" and non-Life, in Povinelli's terms: time that reads the relation between humans and between the environment and humans within vast, intergenerational, epi(stemi)c time frames. In this respect, one could argue that, while non-Aboriginal cultures may be unaccustomed to grasping Timothy Morton's hyperobjects, for Aboriginal cultures this may indeed be a *customary* activity, consequent upon multigenerational and animist perspectives. Morton defines hyperobjects as "things that are massively distributed in time and space relative to humans" (2013, 1), his exemplary hyperobject being global warming.[6]

The opening of *Carpentaria* is radical in its displacement of humans from the forefront of characterization in the novel. It begins with the Rainbow serpent who carves the valleys and the rivers of the area and then takes up residence in the limestone aquifers it has molded. However, the serpent is not contained; it is not *in* the environment of the Gulf; it *is* that environment: "This is where the giant serpent continues to live deep down under the ground in a vast network of limestone aquifers. They say its being is porous; it permeates everything. It is all around the atmosphere and it is attached to the lives of the river people like skin" (2). In this sense, the serpent is not an environment so much as it is the very *fabric* of geobiographical being, in which the scale of human life is miniscule, and in which humans can live only if they have intimate knowledge of the river, as Normal Phantom does:

> It takes a particular kind of knowledge to go with the river, whatever its mood. It is about there being no difference between you and the movement of the water as it seasonally shifts tracks according to its own mood. A river that spurns human endevour on one dramatic gesture, jilting a lover who has never really been known, as it did to the frontier town built on its banks in the hectic heyday of colonial vigour. A town intended to serve as a port for the shipping trade for the hinterland of Northern Australia. (3)

I am not suggesting that what non-Indigenous readers need to do is to garner Indigenous knowledge of a character such as Normal Phantom, because as Alison Ravenscroft points out, this is impossible (2010). In her recounting of Deborah Bird Rose's account of Yarralin *manngyin*—"that which is connected to the flesh and organs and when a person dies and is buried it gets up again"—Ravenscroft dismisses the obvious English strategy of this account, an appeal to "spirit," quoting Bird Rose once again: Spirit "cannot but signal a body-soul dichotomy which is inappropriate to the Yarralin context." Ravenscroft continues: "Translation fails, and into the gap so easily slips our own vocabulary and generic codes: magic and superstition, myth and magic realism. We make others' objects of knowledge magic in a move that paradoxically tames and familiarizes" (216).

This move is accounted for beautifully in Graham Huggan's definition of the postcolonial exotic (2001), and it is certainly not a move I plan to make; that is to say, I am not promoting making Yarralin objects of knowledge "magic," nor suggesting we can know them as the Yarralin do. Ravenscroft closes her article on *Carpentaria* and its critics with the suggestion that the objects of the other inspire terror: "What might be most unbearable before another's objects is one's own necessary and impartial vision" (216–17). One translation of this into the terms of my argument is that the geobiographical, extra-anthropocentric imaginary and its values are at best terrifying and at worst incomprehensible to readers accustomed to the willful ignorance that colonialist-capitalist culture manifests toward the suffering of those refusing its deadly terms, readers simultaneously attuned to anthropocentric value.

We do not have access to the knowledge of Normal Phantom or the objects of *Carpentaria*, but we can trace in these artifacts a critique of the supposedly rational materialism of white colonizer society. Doing so provides at least a profile of what kinds of unbearable knowledges, or ignorance, the nexus of colonialism, capitalism, and whiteness funds, so to speak. The Uptown crew of whites in *Carpentaria*'s town of Desperance is represented by Mayor Stan Bruiser, who states: "If you can't use it, eat it, or fuck it, it's no use to you" (35). "Everyone in town knew how he bragged about how he had chased every Aboriginal woman in town at various times, until he ran them into the ground and raped them" (41). In *Carpentaria*, mining and rape are related violations. This is because capitalist culture, epitomized by Stan Bruiser, is simultaneously a culture of rape. The instrumentalization of objects extends to sexual gratification and includes the unmaking of the raped body as "human" in its objectification: "If you can't fuck *it*," he says, "*it's* no use to you" (emphasis added), exemplifying the link between sexual assault and commodification I explored in detail in the previous chapter.

A key attribute of extra-anthropocentricity is the ability to accrue value to extrahuman, and thus multigenealogical and multigeological frames of time and space reference, values of a kind that would completely mystify Stan Bruiser, with his assumption of value as the ability to produce immediate gratification for *himself*, as the cult of individual self-"improvement" (actually, evidence of the ability of the self to accumulate wealth) according to the capitalist "ethic," is his mantra. (Bruiser was a hawker selling goods at a profit of 300 to 400 percent after cost to remote towns and Aboriginal camps. In the 1970s he picked up a late-night radio tip, put all his money in a tin-pot mining company that struck it rich in Western Australia, and became wealthy overnight.) Let me take you back to the kind of time and space with which *Carpentaria* begins and which provide a startling contrast to Stan's cripplingly limited perspective.

Carpentaria's narrator explains that Desperance was set up as a harbor; but when the serpent in its infinite being caused the waters to recede permanently from the town, it sought a reason for its being, a myth of origins, an instrumentalist reason for being. At first it found this myth in the need to defend against the "yellow peril"; subsequently, the townsfolk turned to the management of Aboriginal people as their raison d'être:

> When the yellow peril did not invade, everyone had a good look around and found a more contemporary reason for existence. It meant that the town still had to be vigilant. Duty did not fall on one or two; duty was everyone's business. To keep a good eye out for when the moment presented itself, to give voice to a testimonial far beyond personal experience—to comment on the state of their Blacks. To do so was regarded as an economic contribution to State rights, then, as an afterthought, to maintaining the decent society of the nation as a whole (4).

The association between economic productivity and decency is exemplified in the ways in which the mining company further splits opinion in the Aboriginal community. Some are persuaded by its promise of a secure life; others, like Will Phantom, Normal's son, protest ferociously against the mining company's incursions on and into the land. Standing as woeful testimony to the mine's lack of human right once again is Kevin Phantom, the one who works only one day for the mine, and that day becomes disabled mentally and physically for life, finally being accosted by three white boys in hoods who drag him behind the back of a car.

If the critic Ravenscroft sees Aboriginal objects that are sacred as threatening whites with the insecurity of whites' partial knowledge, it seems clear that, conversely, mining capitalism produces benefits, such as modern housing, that produce fear of their consequences in some Aboriginals wary of the effects of colonial capitalism. Will is an activist against the mine, and old man Joseph Midnight refuses to move into the modern housing provided by the mine altogether.

"This is the only safe place left," old man Joseph Midnight kept repeating to himself, as he wandered in and out of his old bit of a lean-to home. The structure of tin and plastic, in an ongoing state of disarray, stood behind the brand-new house the government had given him free—lock, stock and barrel—for cooperating with the mine, but which he said 'was too good to use.' (369)

Joseph feels he should never have been left, as an old man, to make the decision whether to cooperate with the mine or not: "He spat toward the new house whenever it caught his eye. He was suffering the unrelenting pain of a wrong decision" (372). His only hope for the future (not necessarily his own future defined as the limited world of the currently living, but his hope for a geobiographical future) lies in his love for Will Phantom, his wife Hope, and their child, Bala. When Will goes to sea to find Hope and Bala (who, for those of you who've not read the story, left with Elias, and Elias returns dead, but they don't), old man Joseph Midnight "remembered a ceremony he had never performed in his life before, and now, to his utter astonishment, he passed it on to Will. . . . The song was so long and complicated and had to be remembered in the right sequence where the sea was alive, waves were alive, currents alive, even the clouds." Joseph Midnight warns: "'Will, remember, you will only travel where the sea country lets you through'" (373). Immediately prior to this paragraph, the narrative talks about the "Clayplans [that] breathed like skin, and you could feel it, right inside the marrow of your bones. The old people said it was the world stirring itself, right down to the sea. . . . It made you think that whatever it was living down underneath your feet was much bigger than you" (369).

Carpentaria-land: Introducing Extra-Anthropocentric Human Right-Making

I may risk being read as anthropoligizing the Yarralin and Wright's narrative, but let me go so far as to say that this is an animist cosmology, in which the skin of the earth and the skin of the people are connected. The connection is not spiritual in the Cartesian sense of the word, but embodied: remember that you can live with the river of the opening scenes of *Carpentaria* (quoted above) only if you can breathe as slowly as it does, if you can imagine your subjectivity and that of your land as one and the same through the lens of geobiographical time. I agree with Ravenscroft that we cannot know what this might mean to a person of the Yarralin; but this does not mean we can't open ourselves up to the horror that old man Joseph Midnight sees in the "normal" vision of mining housing. The movement for environmental justice addresses issues of the contamination of the poor in the service of the wealthy. The direction I wish to go in, rather, is to ask: what if the notion of geobiographical time were perceived *not* as a threat to the living human, but rather, contra Morton, as an *integral part of* extra-anthropocentric quotidian being? What if, instead, ignorance of geobiographical time results in horror not only in terms of our ability to understand the necessary conditions for ecological well-being, but also in terms of colonizer-capitalist ignorance of human well-being as it might be (re)articulated in human rights within a geobiographical framework: extra-anthropocentric human-rightness?

This may be hard to imagine, because settler culture tends to fear it is as a speck of dust in the realms of geobiographical time, and accordingly, we tend to imagine that accruing subjectivity to the environment geobiographically conceived, and to us geobiographically conceived, would result in the diminishment of the human, much as a landscape of grandeur diminishes the human subjects painted small within it—this would be the extra-anthropocentric as Morton's hyperobject. Yet, if its skin is our skin, somehow—perhaps we don't need to know *how* this might be to at least investigate this possibility—then is such diminishment even rational, let alone inevitable? What if the diminishment of the land's rights (an example from *Carpentaria* would be the poisoning of land and the rivers, and thus the kingfishers, through the mine's production of lead waste) is indeed an attack on *human* understandings of rightness, in a kind of hyper-intersubjectivity? This is of course more possible to consider in theory than in practice. In practice, the imperative to produce goods in a material system that is itself always hungry, that is by the logic of surplus goods and labour *never* satiable, cannot enable the kinds of human rights we might begin to envision with reference to the values of geobiographical time, because rights within a geographical framework would need to assume sustainability as part and parcel of a multigenerational/sustainable ethic.

In a 1990s essay entitled "Do Rocks Listen?" that deals with the challenges of Aboriginal land-claims rights in Australia, Povinelli stages the incomprehension of a land-claims judge listening to Betty Billawag explain the importance of a nearby Dreaming site, Old Man Rock. Betty Billawag explains that Old Man Rock "listened to and smelled the sweat of Aboriginal as people as they passed by hunting, gathering, camping, or just mucking about. She outlined the importance of such human-Dreaming/environmental interactions to the health and productivity of the countryside" (505). A companion of Povinelli's points out to her (Povinelli) that the judge doesn't seem to believe Betty Billawag's animist "knowing" that Old Man Rock is a subjective witness; Povinelli responds that she thinks the judge believes that Betty Billawag believes what she herself, Betty, is saying; he just doesn't believe it *himself*. Povinelli then goes on to say that the courts have accrued value to "traditional" beliefs and practices of the Aboriginals by splitting these off from their referents. In other words, such traditional practices are a compromise in an overarching value system that places capitalist value as the norm(al) and therefore invisible and unassailable belief that can then "afford" to make accommodations for traditional claims, but only where and when such claims do not undermine productivity in terms of the Australian gross domestic production. Here Australian Aboriginal labor is accommodated but does not stand on its own terms. "While belief and value, or more exactly, divergent epistemologies and the socioeconomic and legal apparatuses that support them, are at the heart of the conflict, Western economy and its epistemologies have been miraculously separated from the discussion. *Western beliefs are not on the examining table*" (514).

So here, then, is the challenge. If Betty Billawag needs to outline her belief/value system for the scrutiny of a court that sees no reason to put its own settler-colonialist-capitalist values under scrutiny, how can I, in my reading of *Carpentaria*, restage this confrontation differently? Here the difference consists in, first, having terms for acknowledging Aboriginal extra-anthropocentric labor and, second, not "outsourcing" responsibility for extra-anthropocentric human rightness to Aboriginal animist communities, who have (long) been burdened with the radical incommensurability of extra-anthropocentric being and colonial capitalism.

Phantom Labor: Extra-Anthropocentric Human Right-making

First, I'd like to suggest that the persistence depicted in *Carpentaria*, particularly in its representations of art-making, demonstrates how much labor goes into contesting and surviving the make-work project of settler-colonial capitalism. Settler-colonial capitalism works within what Povinelli calls "the carbon imaginary": its logic is that not only of consumption of carbon-based fuels but also, as Povinelli points out, of fundamental acceptance of distinctions between carbon-based life forms as living and others as dead (2014). What we need to rethink radically, she suggests, is the divisions between the living and the nondead (because that which is nondead is not, has not been, and never will be able to be alive in the terms of the carbon imaginary). Thus, it is the assemblage of the geological and the biological that forms Wright and Povinelli's mutual insistence on building geobiographical imaginaries that question the very notions of life and finitude that undergird Western philosophy. One way in which we can ground this concept is in the forms of art-making we find in *Carpentaria*. The novel figures intergenerational exchanges not only as interhuman, but as decimating Povinelli's geontology. In her 2017 *Geontologies*, Povinelli defines geontological power as that which neoliberal governance uses to determine distinctions between Life and non-Life. According to Robin Wright, Povinelli explores how "late liberalism uses different ontologies of human and nonhuman arrangements of existence to both celebrate and discredit certain economic and cultural practices in order to facilitate the entwined logics of extractive capital and settler liberalism" (2017). One can think of *Carpentaria*'s art as the opposite of Povinelli's geontological power, as a set of relations not only between generations of persons but also between the *bios* and the *geos*, the living and the not-dead, over time. This is the art of the novel as geobiography. Further, while intergenerational, geobiographical relations are marked by mutual obligation, they are also marked by gift exchange. Thus old man Joseph Midnight gives Will his boat, knowing that he will not survive to see Will return it, and he himself receives the gift of the stories and rituals he uses to prepare Will for his journey. Perhaps the preeminent geobiographical artistic capacity is given to Normal Phantom (and, on occasion, withdrawn from him): he can take the bodies and bones of dead fish and reincarnate them so that they sparkle with a vivacity that has nothing to do with taxidermy. The fish embody the vivacity of the dead who are marked not only as sites of mourning but also as sites of the celebration of the undead. This is highlighted by their capacity to sing from the walls of Normal's fish room, his studio, where they are kept. Indeed, *Carpentaria*, as Ravenscroft notes, is marked by characters not knowing who is dead and who is alive, with cross-dressings of the dead as alive and the live as dead. This radical de-categorization, or rather *dis*categorization, marks the importance of the artistry required to navigate the fabric *between* the geo- and bio-spheres, artistry that partakes of the persistence in the face of colonial capitalism and its abuses.

The fact that capitalism has no truck with this form of labor—just as it cannot recognize the labor of the Australian Aboriginal Dreaming interface except in terms of liberal accommodation that serves its own ends—can be seen, in the sense of human-rights practices as extra-anthropocentric, as a human-rights violation. The right to interact from and in a geos–bios right-making framework forms the antithesis of what one might call normative, or capital, human rights. Thus, Povinelli points out that, in relation to Aboriginal human-rights claims, in no way has the non-Aboriginal Australian government or public altered its understanding of the factual grounds of work, labor, human subjectivity, or environmental insentience. In short, the state produces a classic Batesian double message. It tells Indigenous persons: "Your beliefs are absolutely essential to your economic well-being; your beliefs make no rational sense in the assessment of your economic well-being" (Povinelli, 1995, 516).

This is a putative separation of labor and culture, with the reification of culture as *not* labor and art as product, rather than productive of resilient relationships in the geontological sense of transactions of obligation and gift. Art-making, in the particular aspect of persistence in which I place the examples from *Carpentaria,* is the making of an alternative extra-anthropocentric human right. It is a space, or an assemblage of materials, carbon and other, where or in which we can recognize, and are recognizing, that what constitutes the human right to live geobiographically is radically undermined in inverse proportion to the exploitation of contested land for capitalist surplus. Such persistence is about the endurance of ways of living that exceed the carbon imaginary and capitalist human rights. Fetishizing Aboriginal resilience in a context in which it is celebrated from the aspect of the separation of what is perceived to be Aboriginal culture, as opposed to productive labor, plays into the liberal governance of Aboriginality criticized by Povinelli, and in some sense naturalizes the notion that Aboriginal culture can withstand, or is resilient to, colonial capitalism, such that non-Aboriginals do not have to take responsibility for colonial capitalism's harms.[7] Instead, I identify the arts of specifically geobiographical persistence as forms of human right-making in practice.

The Bones of *Carpentaria*: Featuring Extra-Anthropocentric Human Right-Making

I propose, then, that there are arts of human right-making that need to be identified *as such* before we can understand what we might be killing off in aligning ourselves with the epistemology of the carbon imaginary and its values. Specifically, late capitalism assigns value differentially across a set of human labors that are positively assessed if they are productive within the terms of the carbon imaginary. They are not only negatively assessed, but *unable to be named*, if they issue from the eruption of Western epistemologies enacted by geobiographical practices. I agree with Ravenscroft that *Carpentaria* presents us with holes in our knowledge that we as non-Aboriginal readers, or more specifically non-Yanyuwa/Waanyi readers, can never fill (2010, 214). However, building on Ravenscroft's argument, and the reading of *Carpentaria* offered here, we can begin to see the profile of the kinds of epistemologies we are as yet only beginning to name. This epistemological "infancy" originates from our difficulty in generating knowledge outside of the fundamental carbon binary of life–death that geobiographical practices fundamentally reject. The presentism of the carbon imaginary is entrenched in and by capitalist interests.

So, how *can* I characterize the extra-anthropocentric human right-making I draw from arts-based practices in *Carpentaria*? First, as noted above, these practices create a radical indeterminacy over the life or death of carbon-based forms. Wright's Normal Phantom has the gift of reanimating the fish; and there are numerous other instances in which we cannot know whether characters are "dead" or "alive," but are forced to reflect on their beings nevertheless. Nor does *Carpentaria* wish to satisfy us about the status of these forms. As Ravenscroft puts it:

> It makes the very division into magical and rational, living and dead, body and country undecidable—at least for this white reader. This is not an undecidability that rests only in the Aboriginal protagonists, as some reviewers have suggested: it's not just Normal Phantom or his son Will who can't always tell what is living and what is dead, what is dream and what is waking, where one's own mind ends and another begins. This undecidability is produced in me too. (2010, 207)

Interestingly, critic Katherine England describes what I am identifying as an imaginative capacity for practicing extra-anthropocentric human rights—that is, the refusal of a carbon imaginary—as an inability, or at least a deficiency. She says Normal Phantom "has difficulty differentiating between dead and living visitors to his fish room" (cited in Ravenscroft

2010, 222). This idea that the refusal of the carbon imaginary represents a lack of expertise may explain the fact that every major publisher in Australia rejected *Carpentaria* until it was published by the independent Giramondo in 2006. The fish withdraw their singing in Normal's studio for periods of time, during which he is unable to undertake his radical "non-taxidermy," but they do not die, in the sense that they come back when they wish to, once again enabling the craft, which is mutually desired by Normal and the fish; otherwise, nothing happens.

Second, this practice of extra-anthropocentric right-making, characterized by the co-constitution of the artist and the environment they both inhabit and shape, renders the art-as-product a term of impossibility. While those who come with their dead fish for Normal to reanimate, in a practice that defies any commonsense notion of taxidermy, may think of the artifact brought forth as products, the fish in Normal's room defy the facticity of deadness: they register the mood of the room, sing in choirs, and "play dead" when Normal loses his capacity to reanimate them temporarily. His art-making is unmistakably related to his knowledge of the seasons, the rivers, and the seas of the area; his arts are co-constitutive of himself and the environment he both inhabits and shapes, and that both inhabits and shapes him. It is not dictated by his clients.

Third, these artistic practices, or rituals, of extra-anthropocentric human right-making are taking place in communities where access to human-rights discourses of the conventional, legal kind are so alien as to be laughable. The icons of the modern nation-state in Wright's *Carpentaria* bear this out, from the mayor with his penchant for raping Aboriginal women to Girlie's preventing Truthful, the policeman, from finding Elias's bones and accusing her father, Normal, of Elias's murder by accepting Truthful's unwanted advances, and thereby distracting him from investigation of the raging fire she and her siblings set precisely to protect their father from such an arrest. They secure Truthful's ignorance and appetites for their own purposes. Normal is frantic when he realizes they have stolen Elias's bones from the fish room and burned them, as the "dead" Elias is Normal's companion in that room. Thus, Truthful's ignorance is not simply lack of knowledge about the origins of the fire and the bones of Elias; it is also his ignorance of the value of those bones to Normal Phantom, a value that Truthful would never be able to fathom in a million years as residing in what would seem to him, and does indeed seem to Normal's daughters, a pile of smelly old bones.

Fourth, these practices are under threat, precisely because, as Povinelli has pointed out, liberal governance entails tolerance in an era of postcolonial, postslavery, and racial recognition; but such recognition and tolerance takes place only within the (il)logic of what liberal governance perceives as productive or sensible, or, I would argue, in Judith Butler's terminology, "speakable" (1997, 132). This is the structure that produces the contradiction whereby Australian liberal governance of difference, as described by Povinelli, enables Aboriginal culture only inasmuch as it recognizes historical modes of being Aboriginal as described by settlers at the time of colonization, and inasmuch as the lands claimed have been occupied continuously by a community whose patriarchy is historically traceable. However, cultural practices that cannot play by these rules are under a death threat, because colonial displacement and genocide make the claim to traditional land and ways of living impossible, and because liberal recognition demands the gold standard of economic productivity, which discounts extra-material meaning. Or, as Povinelli puts it, citing Kristie McClure: "The appropriateness or desirability of toleration" of specific groups assures "a discursive framework within which toleration makes sense"; "many unregulated publics go beyond the conceptual barriers of the frame of toleration, 'beyond which toleration appears foreclosed as senseless, as nonsense, in both principle and practice'" (2006, 13). That *Carpentaria* took so long to be published has in part to do with its discursivity exceeding the framework "beyond which toleration appears foreclosed as senseless").

Apprehension of these artistic practices as human right-making activities enables a language, I propose, that increases our understanding of what liberal toleration not only allows to live and lets die, but what the liberal governance strategies of late colonial capitalism can *make* die. This is the case precisely because we are not accustomed to being able to name these practices in connection with human rights in the first instance, owing to the values of the "human" colonialist-capitalist imaginary subtending contemporary human-rights discourses. Having a language for what's at stake enables humanists to forge alliances with those working across the geos–bios divide in the natural sciences and simultaneously in the countercultures of capitalism actually at work within our communities. This strategy of geobiographical articulation presents itself as an important step in taking a harm-reduction approach to the mastery of carbon-imaginary values, whose prospects for sustainability not only intergenerationally and transnationally, but even in the shorter term and in the first and second worlds, are far more in question than those of the arts of extra-anthropocentric right-making need be.

Conclusion: Novel Writing as Right-Making Practice and Artifact

What, then, has our reading of *Carpentaria* as an extra-anthropocentric human right-making artifact accomplished? It denaturalizes and renders absurd normative human rights by depicting the scene of rights-bearing and rights-seeking subjects as incomprehensible, or comprehensible only within colonialist-capitalist regimes of governance. Further, it articulates the Aboriginal rights-seeking persona of the NTER a fiction, one that is rendered pathological in view of the assumed health of normative, rights-bearing citizens. Self-harming behaviors, such as substance abuse, youth suicide, and related behaviors can be seen in an extra-anthropocentric context not as pathological, but as forms of preemptive harm reduction against colonialist-capitalist uses of what materialist cultures consider the Aboriginal body, but what is actually Aboriginal *being*. Further, *Carpentaria* demonstrates that some of the concepts Morton considers hyperobjects may not originate from an anthropocentrism that is innate to all human subjects, since the narrative poses an extra-anthropocentric hyperintersubjectivity as evidence of Aboriginal geobiographical being. From this perspective, anthropocentric human rights are unsustainable for humans among other beings, and are therefore deadly, or "capital" rights. For example, climate change as a hyperobject may be normative to the "citizen-who-bears-rights," but is really intersubjectively constituted in a geobiographical framework, one that understands the mutual interdependence of humans, nonhuman animals, and other beings. To the extent that the Aboriginal is considered human, bearing in mind that the Aboriginal is human only in terms of liberal accommodation, the human may seem capable of imagining geobiographical frameworks. However, as long as extra-anthropocentric being is recognized only as a Povinellian compromise in an economy of colonialist-capitalist governance, extra-anthropocentric *value* is, in actuality, inaccessible to the rights-bearing and rights-granting human who depends upon such recognition.

If one reads *Carpentaria* as a normative human-rights narrative, it is possible to fetishize normative bearing of human rights, with "fetishism" defined as "that perversion which substitutes a fabricated object for a natural one perceived to be missing" (Suleiman 1990, 148). The fabricated object here, as in the NTER, would be the fantasy of the Aboriginal as seeking conventional rights, since there is no Aboriginal character in *Carpentaria* that trusts national or local governance as a source of rights in the long term. The natural object perceived to be missing would be the rights-bearing Aboriginal subject. Here I have attempted to offer an alternative reading, one that reframes the rather limited role literature is placed in when it is read as formative of normative human rights, or evidence of the failure of normative human-rights regimes to deliver on their promise, or both. *Carpentaria* offers a diagnostic of normative human-rights regimes. It demonstrates both the reason for their failure, which is their dependence on an anthropocentric notion of rights within the liberal politics of recognition, and an alternative to them: not the novel as a genre of the human per se, but the possibility of novel-writing as both practice and artifact of extra-anthropocentric human right-making. This opens up a role for the novel far beyond the horizons of its instrumentality in the service of normative human-rights regimes; the novel becomes a space of extra-anthropocentric human right-making in the sense of right-making creativity. One can affirm this creativity, however, only outside of readings of the tropes of Aboriginal as exotic and the Aboriginal as pathological, an eternally rights-seeking persona in view of the authority of rights-bearing structures of governance. The *value* of extra-anthropocentric right-making in *Carpentaria* thus depends upon the assumption—indeed the presumption—of Aboriginal sovereignty on geobiographically conceived Aboriginal ground. That such grounding may not entail, but decrease, white suffering may be a hyperobjective concept for settlers, but that does not, thankfully, make hyperobjectivity actual.

Afterword

Simultaneous Reading and Slow Becoming

What, one may ask, are the implications of the effluent eye for changing reading practices in the wake of the genre of the human? How might one read in ways that are open to an extra-anthropocentric right-making? It might seem odd to insert an afterword on a practice that I have presumably been exemplifying in the previous five chapters! However, I would like to turn my attention here to how we might read writing—not just *Carpentaria*—in ways that exceed settler time[1] and the genre of the human: What might artifacts look like biogeographically, with an effluent eye?

One of the most persuasive and distinct descriptions of settler time comes from a novel published long before the naming of settler time, at least in scholarly literature. I am writing here of J. M. Coetzee's meditation in his 1980 *Waiting for the Barbarians,* focalized through his protagonist and narrator, a magistrate on a colonial frontier known only as "the Magistrate," on what the state known only as "Empire" has done to time. The Magistrate's reflection comes after he has turned against Colonel Joll, a visiting authority of Empire and expert in torture, whose sojourn on the frontier leads to the imprisonment of the Magistrate and then his abandonment in the small frontier town he used to administrate:

> Calf-deep in the soothing water I indulge myself in the wishful vision. I am not unaware of what such daydreams signify, dreams of becoming an unthinking savage, of taking the cold road back to the capital, of groping my way out to the ruins in the desert, of returning to the confinement of my cell, of seeking out the barbarians and offering myself to them to use as they wish. Without exception they are dreams of ends: dreams not of how to live but of how to die. And everyone, I know, in that walled town sinking now into

darkness (I hear the two thin trumpet calls that announce the closing of the gates) is similarly preoccupied.

What has made it impossible for us to live in time like fish in the water, like birds in air, like children? It is the fault of Empire! Empire has created the time of history. Empire has located its existence not in the smooth recurrent spinning time of the cycle of the seasons but in the jagged time of rise and fall, of beginning and end, of catastrophe. Empire dooms itself to live in history and plot against history. One thought alone preoccupies the submerged mind of Empire: how not to end, how not to die, how to prolong its era. By day it pursues its enemies. It is cunning and ruthless; it sends its bloodhounds everywhere. By night it feeds on images of disaster: the sack of cities, the rape of populations, pyramids of bones, acres of desolation. A mad vision yet a virulent one: I, wading in the ooze, am no less infected with it than the faithful Colonel Joll as he tracks the enemies of Empire through the boundless desert, sword unsheathed to cut down barbarian after barbarian until at last he finds and slays the one whose destiny it should be (or if not his then his son's or unborn grandson's) to climb the bronze gateway to the Summer Palace and topple the globe surmounted by the tiger rampant that symbolizes eternal domination, while his comrades below cheer and fire their muskets in the air. (146)

Here the Magistrate reflects that, even though he has made a stand against Empire through his confrontation of Joll, his position against Empire's abuse of land and fisher-folk and "barbarians" does not amount to a different way of being for the Magistrate. It does not model how he and others like him can envision life outside of the historical trajectory of Empire. While the magistrate calls his embeddedness in Empire a mad vision, he claims that he is no less infected with it than Colonel Joll. What he is infected with, I propose, is the genre of man, the normate, and its entanglement in colonial capitalism. Put bluntly, he doesn't know how to be any other way. He can dream only of ends, he and his colonial-settler compatriots, ends both in the sense of conclusions and terminations and in terms of means to such ends. That is to say, the settler-colonial imagination is programmed toward ends that are always predetermined: accumulation through dispossession and winning the last battle, even though every battle is always potentially the last battle and must be fought accordingly, with no break, no reflection on the lack of change such battles produce, or on the claustrophobic bubble they both create and defend. This seems particularly valent in the United States currently, where the Trump movement and its associated fantasies and nightmares seem symptoms extraordinaire of fear at the prospect of increasingly challenged white supremacy. That there can be no whiteness without its supremacy, and no white life without Black death, is part and parcel of this "mad vision."

Reading outside this imagination requires a radical break in the anthropocentric time and space of empire: the right to imagine an outside of human rights that encompasses right-making. What characterizes colonialist-capitalist time is the notion of the lifespan of the state and its citizens as the only form of being, and even then, only if that being is catalogued. For, just as the Australian state demands that Aboriginal peoples demonstrate ongoing/continuing inhabitance of their land to verify their land claims when conditions of proof are impossible (they have oral and not written stories, and colonization drove them from those lands and created interruption of that inhabitance), in that same way, the state places importance not on its citizens, but on what "it" knows about those citizens: "Whether the subject lives or dies is not a concern of the state. What matters to the state and its records is whether the citizen is alive or dead," says the narrator of another Coetzee novel, *Diary of a Bad Year* (2007, 5). The citizen is no longer a subject, just an object, the knowledge of which is a means to the end of population control, in the sense of surveillance. He has an identity but not a subjectivity, whereas the state takes on subjectivity with no discernable identity.

One could argue that this is Coetzee's Magistrate's "mad . . . yet virulent vision" (1980, 146) taken to the extreme, in that the ability to be a subject is illogically projected onto the state to maintain the state's subjects "on its side," and in the process, subjects are rendered objects. In this sense, the Magistrate does not know how to live other than as abject, since being for or against the state depends on the fiction of the state as a subject capable of mutual constitution between state-as-subject and citizen-as-subject. It also depends on the fiction that being for or against something constitutes a creative introduction of novel forces. However, being against apartheid, for example, is a necessary but insufficient criterion for envisioning a postapartheid world. Strategic essentialism has its limits. What is risky, I suggest, is the acceptance of the fiction of the state as a beneficent or antagonistic subject, rather than a bureaucratic proliferation that operates on the fiction of being capable of mutuality. What happens, however, when Empire loses its clothes?

Living with awareness of the state as a bureaucratic proliferation whose "offer" of mutuality is a guise, creates a crisis for the Magistrate. He can imagine himself only as an abject subject in relation to the state, whose end, envisioned in the slaying of the tiger rampant by the enemy of the state, will mean his end, because it means the end of his raison d'être as normate. In the context of such addiction to colonial histories, one can see that the myth of *terra nullius* is adjunct to the myth of the blank page before writing. The blank page is analogous to the birth of the normate subject, whose will is magically wrought into being either in writing or being written, erasing prior histories of Indigenous being, Indigenous labor, slavery, indentured and other forms of ruthless work, and working conditions that make the myth of the blank page possible—the slash-and-burn clearing of the forest, as it were, to make the clearing from which the blank page issues.

Yet, if we collect the threads of each of the previous chapters, a different subjectivity becomes possible from that of the liberal individual, the normate, the "human" in Sylvia Wynter's "genre of man," who writes his own ticket. First, we can read with the simultaneity of human generations in play: ancestor-living-yet-to-be-born. In this instance, we might apprehend an aesthetic narrative that centers storytelling that keeps open the pathways between the unborn, living, and ancestors, much as Wole Soyinka's groundbreaking *Death and the King's Horseman*, Es'kia Mphahlele's African humanism, Alexis Wright's *Carpentaria*, and Masande Ntshanga's *The Reactive* enact such openings. All draw attention to openings through the aspect of ritual. In this sense, we might think of ourselves as readers not as, but akin to, old man Joseph Midnight, who remembers "a ceremony he had never performed in his life before, and now, to his utter astonishment, he passed it on to Will. . . . The song was so long and complicated and had to be remembered in the right sequence where the sea was alive, waves were alive, currents alive, even the clouds" (Wright 2006, 360). This takes us to the biogeographical space where, as Joseph Midnight warns Will, he "will only travel where the sea country lets you through" (360). The repetition of remembering can be read here in the simultaneity of the presence of the ancestors, living and unborn, as the dismembering of the human-as-subject and the remembering of the human-as-co-constitutive of the "environment," not as an array of objects for extractive industry, but as they to whom Will must listen and with whom he must negotiate for their mutual well-being. The sea, the waves, the currents, and even the clouds are *alive*. This is not a reading in which the end of the novel coincides with the end of the simultaneous interrelationships iterated by the narrative; the narrative is an opportunity to remember and exemplify the simultaneous co-constitution of extra-anthropocentric being. The page was/is never blank and we-it-they was/is always there as an opportunity, as a ritual in need of practice.

The critical reading of the colonial in Western medicine reminds us that the constitution of the self as healthy in relation to the diseased other produces suffering, as does the simple reversal of this formulation; it reminds us that this is entangled with the assumption of Western medical conventions as healthy and all others as superstition. What the unreliability of these oppositional structures means in relation to co-constituted subjectivity is that we cannot compose the other as a knowing and knowable set of knowledges, embodiments, and attitudes that we merely have to inhabit to magically become that subjectivity. As Ravenscroft reminds us in relation to the Yarralin *manngyin*, "we make others' objects of knowledge magic in a move that paradoxically tames and familiarizes" when we think we can simply shift into liberal recognition of those objects within the framework of the postcolonial exotic. What is required is first a recognition that *the other as such does not exist*: there is no amalgamation of otherness to the self of the genre of the human that makes sense. I am therefore not claiming in any way that African humanism and Waanyi being are fixed in time, interchangeable, or objects to be known, even able to be known, by the white reader. I am suggesting that they are openings whose performance in narrative ritualizes the invitation to realize the being-together they offer. This being-together requires both the patience of a Lindanathi in *The Reactive*, a patience to wait/be with, rather than to intervene to restore a putative genre of the human, and a receptiveness to bearing mutual if imperfect witness, rather than an occupation of "the other." Disease is seen to be a deficit within the genre of man: they who do not conform to that genre are "naturally" ill, most spectacularly if they have broken the covenant: that belief in the genre of man and that its liberal-human practices offers a "way up." This is the sleight of hand in which illness produces nonconformity to the genre of the human, just as the genre itself produces its "others" as ill. The trope of "tropical medicine" speaks to the remedy for decadence being a raid on the frontier. What this does is detract enormously from wellness as a mutually constitutive set of practices. It is reduced instead to the clinical scene of intervention as the magic bullet. In this respect, being with the nonhuman animals who may harbor and transmit Covid-19, for example, will tell us not only what animal or set of animals the virus came from, but more importantly, what practices led to our human–animal vulnerability, as such practices are likely to be the source of the next viral wave. Fifth-wave public-health theory is much more likely to be a comprehensive tool for community health in the future than "personalized medicine," defined as "an emerging practice of medicine that uses an individual's genetic profile to guide decisions made in regard to the prevention, diagnosis, and treatment of disease" (National Human Genome Research Center n.d.)

Chapter 3 proposes that we can critically approach the settler-colonial relation to the genre of the human as an addiction. One of the points of this chapter is that settler colonialists do not tend to think of themselves as deprived; nor, in the decolonial context, do anti-colonials think of settler-colonials as deprived. Yet I think of settler-colonials as deprived differently from colonialist-capitalists' "others" in relation to liberal governance, as the comparison between the novels of Haigh and Ntshanga suggests. To be motivated to believe in the colonialist-capitalist state, to believe that there is no "outside" to that state, produces what we might call the pathology of acquisition as both fetish and addiction: the material goods do not produce everything humans require in the alignment of stuff and body as object, and self and mind as subject. This puts figures like the three glue-sniffing youths of *Carpentaria* into the position of harm reduction. While some may argue that they "choose" to sniff glue, thus demonstrating the resilience of the liberal human as mastering the world through individual choice, this "choice" is not choice, but a secondary effect of living under conditions of extreme structural violence, as highlighted by the case of Kevin Phantom in *Heat and Light*. The addiction to beginnings and endings, and to acquisition and consumption, is proposed as answering an urge to fill the existential gap created by the Cartesian split, an urge to ward off fears of invasion and death, but Kevin's story exposes that urge as an ongoing and repeated failure to win or be satiated, since the extreme of bubble safety is never safe, or safe enough.

When I worked on the material that forms the ground of chapter 4, on sexual assault, I received specific criticism for applying a harm-reduction lens to gender-based violence (GBV) in the rural areas, such as encouraging networks of women to stay in touch though cell-phone networks and to text one another if they knew they were entering dangerous territory with partners or other community members. They developed a set of strategies like calling the texter for help or to borrow some sugar, or to come to an "emergency" women's church meeting. I never understood the lack of practicality that critics of harm reduction in contexts of GBV seemed to embody: the idea that, because there should be no GBV, there should be no harm-reduction strategy. Such a strategy, they imply, would somehow "suggest" that GBV is ok because we would be working toward reduction rather than simply demanding eradication. Yet the denial of harm reduction is a way of outsourcing GBV without any intervention in communities without resources; and it's a way of saying that any search for resources that does not result in the elimination of GBV forever and everywhere immediately falls short of the mark and is therefore somehow unethical. The practice of simultaneous reading teaches us that this is not so. If colonial reading is about linearity, anticolonial reading is about simultaneity. Aboriginal peoples can be in the state of colonization but have a sense of their co-constituted subjectivity as that which exceeds this time, into seven generations "before" and "after" now, and exceeds the current "landscape" as well, into decolonized relations with what we call the "environment," through various practices and rituals, rural, urban, and in-between. Mphahlele's African humanism also requires such simultaneous reading in its commitments to the unborn, the living, and the ancestors.

Simultaneous reading, however, is not the property of all those who are "others" to Western culture, as though they were all one and the same and interchangeable: the Other, the Indian, and the Black come into being only as spurious amalgamations necessitated by settler-colonial and colonialist-capitalist tunnel vision in their joint racism. Indeed, simultaneous reading cracks open the paradigm of the Other, insisting on the importance of simultaneous differences, not the binary. As Éduoard Glissant puts it, "the West is not in the West. It is a project, not a place" (1989, 52)—a project of normate, biopolitical subject-making.

With simultaneous reading, we can start to think about a nonlinear imaginary in which we can hold that there should be no structural violence (racism, GBV, ableism, etc.), while *at the same time* making communal efforts to reduce the harms of colonial capitalism. In extreme cases, harm reduction might mean slow death, as in the case of the youths of *Carpentaria*; but in others, it can mean slow becoming. In this sense, harm reduction does not mean "giving in," but creating microgeobiographies of livability, in which slow death does not always win against slow becoming. I do not mean this proposal to replicate the notion of telling the poor that they will be rich in the next life as a tool of making material deprivation palatable; nor am I saying that the marginalized are so resilient that they survive and overcome structural violence. I am saying that the binaries of illness and health and living and dying are not opposites, but a continuum within a frame that enables simultaneous reading as persistence. We can admit the GBV that is right in front of us, in us, and around us, for example, without conceptualizing such acknowledgment as defeat. We need not to suppress GBV through judgment; we can do harm reduction while at the same time being faithful to a vision of a geobiography that does not support GBV as a sustainable practice. *Simultaneous reading is, then, the very epitome of sustainability.* It does not suggest denial of current violence, but it equally does not predict suffocation in the bubble. In many cases, it enables an engagement with the here and now that can be, simultaneously, a substantive contribution to a different geobiography. It is a place of slow becoming, both in its multiple temporalities that take energy to navigate, as Will navigates the sea, and in its multiple achievements, which are the opposite of Morton's hyperobjects. In any case, these achievements are not objects, but co-constitutive collaborations, and their naming as yet often eludes those of us inured to the grammar of colonial capitalism precisely because they are unrecognizable as valuable within that sphere and may be toxic to it.

The idea that what drives sexual assault is settler capitalism and state interests in it, as enunciated by Wright and Million, instead of individualized and racialized pathologies, is just one such observation that escapes visibility. In particular, the fact that the naming of Indigenous victimhood within a global economy of trauma takes place within the same sphere in which appeals for Indigenous sovereignty are heard may well place the realization of the desired sovereignty beyond grasp. "The international law that enables Indigenous trauma to appeal for justice is the same sphere in which we articulate political rights as polities with rights to self-determination. I don't see these as necessarily compatible projects," Million argues (2013, 3). Indeed, it is the very instantiation of the child, the Aboriginal, the Black as victim that is liberal humanism's indexing of its "generosity" in a rhetoric of conjoined apostrophe, pathology, and apology. Million's rejection of the Canadian Truth and Reconciliation Commission's reduction of colonial harm to the period of residential schools and the children abused there, and of healing the traumas of colonization through the individualized care of survivors through individual Western trauma models, points to the inadequacy of the liberal, individual trajectory to "rehabilitation": it is an obstacle to Indigenous health and sovereignty. Instead, Million draws on Indigenous feminist models that deploy what I call simultaneous reading to intervene in settler-colonial pathologizing of Indigenous peoples as perpetual "victims." Million describes a process of "(Un)making the Biopolitical Citizen" (146), which Dara Culhane describes as Million "push[ing] toward collective and politicized movements for healing in everyday lives and in political structures, and against individualized, privatized, and medicalized strategies" (2015, 401). How could this be toxic to the state and its colonialist-capitalist structures? Simultaneous reading enables us to ask questions like: If the invitation to minorities to instantiate themselves as victim-survivors extended by the nation-state and the U.N. discourse is a strategy of continued pathologizing, may not the very recognition received by those the state purports to benefit under normative human-rights regimes indeed be traumatic to those same (supposed) beneficiaries? Here traumatic would not mean the instantiation of the individual citizen as traumatized. Knitting together Million's observations and my conclusions, we can see instead the structural violence that colonial capitalism and its associated rights regimes inflict on apparent beneficiaries. In a cumulative sense, the capitalization of objects and humans as extractive resources cannot hide the toll on the co-constituted subject of human–nonhuman–animal–geological life in all the complexity of that damage. Slow becoming as harm reduction disarms the despair, on one hand, and cynicism, on the other, that encourage and enable "self"-harm of our co-constituted subjectivity through its Cartesian disambiguation. To refuse simultaneous reading as a neocolonial appropriation of "the other" is to fall back on the concept that, if those "normates" the genre of the human purports to serve dream of any other way of being, this is a disavowal of privilege and benefit. Within a simultaneous reading of it, however, if "normates" don't envision slow becoming as an antidote to extractive production, their supposed gains will themselves render the genre of the human a threatened species, not because of poetic justice, but because we can attain sustainability only through the co-constitutive subjectivities of slow becoming. It is not "A Requiem to Late Liberalism" (Povinelli 2016) that is called for, I suggest, so much as an affirmation of slow becoming, with communal refusals to outsource safety to the neoliberal state. Normal Phantom and his singing-fish model presents an aesthetic trajectory for the process. The fish die within normate readings that mark confusions between biological life and death as incapacity; we slowly become when we experience this joining not as confusion, but as artfully curated contingency and propinquity, capable of offering the transiently realized but nevertheless dependable pleasures of slow becoming.

Notes

Positive Country

1. I was motivated by my anger at the U.S. Senate's (happily now abandoned) policy of ABC—Abstain, Be faithful, Condomize—in its approach to HIV prevention in sub-Saharan Africa (SSA). Abstinence may not be possible and/or desirable; women may be faithful, but their partners may well not be, especially in the context of migrant labor systems; and women are not usually empowered to enjoin the use of the male condom (the female condom not having been provided or even available in many areas of the SSA countries).

2. A camp or holding pen for animals, surrounded by a secure protective fence made of thorn bushes.

3. This phenomenon is so widespread as to be ubiquitous, and therefore perversely complex to annotate. A good starting point would be Hund and Mills 2016; the South African iteration usually references the Chacma Baboon (see, for example, Debut 2015). On the complex engagement between Black and white participants in South Africa's Truth and Reconciliation Commission over nonhuman animals, including baboons, see the chapter in Jolly 2010 entitled "Going to the Dogs" (53–81).

4. For a history of Alan Taylor, see Noble 2013. For an exploration of pollution in Wentworth, see Chari 2013.

Introduction

1. Ince's volume contains much more on colonial capitalism, and for excellent work on relations between capitalism and settler colonialism, see Veracini 2015.

2. Veracini, too, is insistent on the present of the settler colonial age, as the title of his book states. He asserts that "settler colonialism makes sense especially if it is understood globally, and that we live in a settler colonial global present" (2015, 53).

3. I use scare quotes around "environment" when I mean it to refer not to the Man-centered concept of environment with a big E, but do not when I intend it to be part of the co-constituted subject: human, nonhuman animal, and environment.

4. For excellent writing on such love, see Simpson 2013.

5. GHRVs are defined by the Human Rights Commission of the Unite Nations as "torture and cruel, inhuman and degrading treatment or punishment, summary and arbitrary executions, disappearances, arbitrary detentions, all forms of racism, racial discrimination and apartheid, foreign occupation and alien domination, xenophobia, poverty, hunger and other denials of economic, social and cultural rights, religious intolerance, terrorism, discrimination against women and lack of the rule of law" (U.N. World Conference on Human Rights in Vienna 1993). The term was used relatively early to critique apartheid (partially explaining the full adoption of the term by South Africa's Truth and Reconciliation Commission): the 1967 U.N. Resolution 1235 of the Economic and Social Council (ECOSOC) compelled the U.N. Commission "to examine information relevant to gross violations of human rights, as exemplified by the policy of apartheid" (Limon and Power 2014, 5). GHRVs would appear not so much to qualify HRVs in terms of relative harm, but rather in terms of clusters of violations that indicate structural rather than interpersonal violence. On the variability of the definition of GRHVs, see Liwanga 2015.

6. See, for example, Coetzee 1982, on "Idleness," and Povinelli 1995, on White Australian ignorance of Aboriginal labor, discussed later in chapter 5. One way of ignoring contemporary Aboriginal presence is to suggest that the Khoi/Inuit/"Indian" "belongs" only in the past and is therefore out of place in metropolitan settings such as universities: a reality that redounds further burdens on Indigenous subjects who work as professionals. See, for example, "This Beautiful Disaster" in Simpson's 2013 *Islands of Decolonial Love*.

7. *Hypercapitalism* is defined as a "term used by Marxist scholars, in their continuing critique of political economy, to depict a relatively new form of capitalistic social organization marked by the speed and intensity of global flows that include exchange of both material and immaterial goods, people, and information. Hypercapitalism, sometimes referred to as 'corporate capitalism,' is blamed by critical scholars for causing misbalance and fragmentation of social life by allowing commercial or business interests to penetrate every aspect of human experience. In other words, critical scholars believe that once-separate spheres of culture and commerce now overlap and that, in return, culture and the way of life in a hypercapitalist society becomes subsumed by the commercial sphere." (Vujnovic 2017).

8. For more on persistence, see Eubanks 2019, 4–7.

9. See, for just two examples, Robertson and Henderson's brilliant 2010 graphic novel, *7 Generations,* and Ruffo's 2010 film *A Windigo Tale*.

10. "Choice disabled" is the term Neil Andersson uses to disavow the kind of body-snatching in which the person who cannot choose (not to be raped, in this case, but the term is one I extend to those not able to eat healthy food owing to

cost, etc.) has choice bestowed theoretically on them to "prove" that individual so-called bad choices are the reason for ill health (2006, 1–3).

1. Effluence, "Waste," and African Humanism

1. In Jolly and Fyfe (2018), we deal extensively with the question of the shortcomings of new materialism in relation to both the questions of deconstructing the liberal human-subject and the question of human rights. Suffice it to say, for the moment, that my critique of the new materialism is based on, first, a denial or ignorance of earlier traditions of African and Indigenous animisms and, second, a focus on the "object's" agency, rather than human capacity for interrelationality with the "objects" of new materialism.

2. Lazarus is referring to the fascination many postcolonial critics of the 1980s and 1990s had with texts that evaded a realist form. Exemplary texts here would be Salman Rushdie's *Midnight's Children*, J. M. Coetzee's *Foe*, and Wilson Harris's *Guyana Quartet*, to name a representative few. Perhaps indicative of this tension is the discussion between David Attwell and Denita Parry in Attridge and Jolly 1998 concerning Coetzee's supposed abstraction.

3. In this respect I agree with Butler and Gambetti and Sabsay that the human rights framework can devalue modes of resistance within the populations it designates vulnerable (2016, 6). What I do not see in Butler's work on vulnerability and resistance, however, is an imaginative reenvisioning of the genre of the human, with which the "presumptive framework" of human rights is so deeply entangled, as I shall argue presently.

4. I am aware of the rejections of resilience as a neoliberal tool for the governance and maintenance of the impoverished at the level of subjects and the "developing" state in Neocleous 2013 and Bracke 2016. I use "persistence" to mean that the precarious, or more inclusively, the effluent, have resources their wealthier counterparts do not have and that the effluent do not have to "give" these resources, which in this case are not objects per se. I also thank my colleague, Charlotte Eubanks (2019) for our conversations about persistence.

5. I understand global capitalism to encompass a broad-spread belief in competitive capitalism as necessity, rather than a chosen way of sociopolitical organization. I also associate capitalism with modes of governance that, whether nationalist or pro-multinational capital flows, see government in the first instance as chief assistant to capitalist industry, not as protector of a range of citizens' rights, not limited to the right to work and/or accumulate capital—that is, as simply protector of the producer-as-consumer.

6. I discuss Berlant's theory at length in chapter 3, where I focus on issues of substance use.

7. This is a version of Arendt's paradox that, to be protected as a citizen, one

has to have the protection of the state, but those who require the protection of citizenship are the stateless: "If a human being loses his political status, he should, according to the implications of the inborn and inalienable rights of man, come under exactly the situation for which the declarations of such general rights provided. Actually, the opposite is the case. It seems that a man who is nothing but a man has lost the very qualities that make it possible for other people to treat him as a fellow-man" (1976, 300).

8. I recognize that I am entertaining a very specific reading here of both Mphahlele and his African humanism, and do not have the scope here to rehearse the exhaustive body of literature written on either African humanism or specifically Mpahelele's version of it. For further reference, see Obee 1999 and Mphahlele 1962; 2002.

9. There is an extent to which my argument here may be seen to resemble that of Karen Barad, who claims that "language has been granted too much power" (2003, 801). However, the focus on representation to the exclusion of the subjectivity of matter is not a global phenomenon. There are cultures, including cultures of the effluent, in which matter has *never stopped* being "substance in its intra-active becoming—not a thing, but a doing, a congealing of agency" (822). The primacy of cultural representation that obscures matter is not a universal phenomenon. Barad implies as much when, citing Joseph Rouse, she describes representationalism as a Cartesian byproduct: the Cartesian legacy proposes that we have more direct access to our thoughts than to the things "outside" us (806). Yet, once again, the Cartesian legacy is not every culture's legacy. Further, I do not use the language of posthumanism, since its understanding of racism is insufficient. While posthumanism understands the importance of racist thought in the establishment of the "human," as Jackson puts it: "I wonder if posthumanists are willing to go one step beyond a critique of the discourse of 'primitivity' by also engaging the knowledge production of those deemed primitive?" (2013, 681).

10. African humanism's overwhelming choice of pronoun is masculine. One has to be careful about reading too much into this, however, as many African languages, including isiZulu, do not have pronouns that indicate gender.

11. This set of beliefs is commonly held, as Mphahlele evidences. Perhaps the most cited reference in this regard is Soyinka's 1976 *Myth, Literature and the African World*.

12. On the issue of the unborn in relation to abortion, Butler argues that "it is not possible to base arguments for reproductive freedom, which include rights to abortion, on a conception of what is living and what is not" (2009, 18).

13. Here I am using the figure of the placenta against itself, as metonymy, like metaphor, is a figure of speech. I am using the word in the sense of a material part of the subject, not in the sense of a representation of such a materiality.

14. Yet not with the inhuman, owing to my reenvisioning of human rights as nonanthropocentric practices of rightness.

15. This was in 1995, and still some time before the domination of the HIV sensibility my generation later experienced, in which HIV was an environment and not an event, as I noted in the preface.

16. Samin interviewed Mphahlele in 1995, and Mphahlele was unable to write his proposed fiction, discussed with Samin, before his death in 2008. I like to think of this prospective fiction as an unborn subject.

17. Apartheid encouraged the "tribalization" of African languages through a fetishized attachment of them to the notorious and deceptively named "homelands" to which it relegated the Black population. This factor, together with the use of English in the relatively liberal mission schools for Blacks, and the imposition of Afrikaans as the medium of instruction for state-run Black schools (the impetus for the Soweto schoolchildren's riots of 1976), contributed to the choice of English over Indigenous languages for Black literary production in South Africa.

18. In his *Phenomenology of Spirit,* Hegel infamously relegates Africa, particularly sub-Saharan Africa, to the realm of the "unhistorical," as it is "undeveloped land" that remains "enmeshed in the natural spirit" (1977, 190). In this sense, Africa would never have been considered a contender in Hegel's master–slave dialectic outlined in the above work. While there are many readings of racism in Hegel, an astute analysis of his treatment of Africa in his *Lectures on the Philosophy of World History* (1837) remains that of Ronald Kuykendall 1993.

19. "Coffin fly" is a generic name for several species of flies that arrive in sequence to feed on decaying flesh and to lay their eggs in the corpse, which provides food for their offspring. It should be noted that these flies are not selective; they feed on many kinds of materials other than corpses but are adept at getting into sealed spaces holding decaying matter, like coffins.

20. From 2001 until 2006 Stephen Lewis worked as the United Nations special envoy for HIV/AIDS in Africa. His task, which he effected with deep commitment, was to draw attention to the HIV/AIDS epidemic and convince leaders and the public of their responsibility in curtailing it.

21. For more on Mbeki's AIDS denialism, see the final chapter of Jolly 2010.

2. Effluence in Disease

1. While the link provided in the bibliography that originally accessed this page now accesses amended material for 2022, the same elements are still there in substance, if not identical in form. The two quotes from WHO that follow are mentioned as is in the 2022 link, apart from the deletion of "AIDS" in the second one.

2. For the figure of the zombie as both consumer-duppy and embodiment of the failure of advanced capitalism, see Lauro and Embry 2008; Moreman 2011; Sutherland and Swan 2011; Lauro 2011a, 2011b; Boluk and Lenz 2011.

3. The more recent link (2014) at cdc.gov/nchhstp/socialdeterminants reads rather differently: "Social determinants of health (SDOH) are the nonmedical factors that influence health outcomes. They are the conditions in which people are born, grow, work, live, and age, and the wider set of forces and systems shaping the conditions of daily life. As defined by the World Health Organization these forces (e.g., racism, climate) and systems include economic policies and systems, development agendas, social norms, social policies, and political systems."

4. This aporia is highlighted by Anderson 1998, Bleakley, Brice Brown, and Bligh 2008, and Jolly 2016.

5. The most recent and useful discussion of this is in the essays in Butler, Gambetti, and Sabsay 2016.

6. This is an all-but-direct quotation from Harraway, except that I have substituted virus–human for dog–human. The original reads: "How might an ethics and politics of significant otherness be learned from taking the dog-human relationships seriously? And, how might stories about dog-human worlds finally convince brain-damaged Americans, and maybe less historically challenged people, that history matters in naturecultures?" (2003, 3). I have excluded the term "brain-damaged" because, while the American exceptionalism to which Harraway refers is extant and well, her terms for referencing it are not mine. In fact, there may well be *clinically* brain-damaged Americans who understand the history of naturecultures better than their fellow citizens without clinical disability.

7. In particular, Paul Farmer's work on Haiti (2006, 2011) is notable for its connection of structural violence to health outcomes. In my introduction I have attempted to supplement his work by first clearly defining structural violence in health-care settings in terms of Johan Galtung's original introduction of the subject (1969) and then locating that term in the context of the contemporary outcomes of colonialist-capitalist violence in terms of the Warwick Research Collective's definition of combined and uneven development (2015).

8. In some sense, a posthuman reading is impossible, as such a reading carries its own utopian bent: how can humans extract themselves from a reading of anything, let alone the entanglements of human migrations and disease? Further, if one understands that the apex of anthropocentric power accrues its benefits differentially through place, race, and space, as it were, the notion that we should now become posthuman, before anthropocentric human's others (female, Black, LBGT, of the global South) have been accorded their "anthropocentric" right, dodges the ethical conundrum of combined but unequal development far too nicely.

9. The Krio ("Creole") comprise African American, West Indian, and liberated African-originating peoples of Sierra Leone.

10. The name "Maroon," according to Merriam-Webster, is probably from French *maron, marron* (*feral, fugitive*), and modification of American Spanish *cimarrón* (*wild, savage*). *Oxford English Dictionary* confirms this origin from *marron* (*feral*) and *cimarrón* (*wild*). Generally, the term refers to descendants of escaped slaves from the West Indies, specifically Jamaica. The Maroons fought two wars against British incursion in the eighteenth century, both ending with treaties being signed between the British and the Maroons.

11. As first reported in *The Washington Post* and later by NBC, President Trump grew frustrated with lawmakers in the Oval Office when they discussed protecting immigrants from Haiti, El Salvador, and African countries as part of a bipartisan immigration deal, according to several people briefed on the meeting. "Why are we having all these people from shithole countries come here?" Trump asked, according to these people, referring to countries mentioned by the lawmakers. Trump then suggested that the United States should instead bring more people from countries such as Norway. In addition, the president singled out Haiti, telling lawmakers that immigrants from that country must be left out of any deal, these people said. "Why do we need more Haitians?" Trump said, according to people familiar with the meeting. "Take them out" (Vitali, Hunt, and Thorp 2018).

12. Cholera is a bacterium, not a virus, but I note it here as yet another instance of disease introduction in the wake of humanitarian intervention.

13. Weheliye points to the obscured element of race in Agamben's overlooking of the *Musselman* as the term used for both women and men followers of Islam.

14. See U.S. DHHS, Office of Minority Health (OMH), n.d.a. Also using the "consumer" language, OMH n.d.b merges various definitions together to state that *culture* is the blended patterns of human behavior that include "language, thoughts, communications, actions, customs, beliefs, values, and institutions of racial, ethnic, religious, or social groups," *cultural competence* is "a set of congruent behaviors, attitudes, and policies that come together in a system, agency, or among professionals that enables effective work in cross-cultural situations," and *competence* in the term *cultural competence* implies that an individual or organization has the capacity to function effectively "within the context of the cultural beliefs, behaviors, and needs presented by consumers and their communities." Material from the OMH n.d.b can also be found through the National Institute of Health at www.ncbi.nlm.nih.gov/books/NBK248431/, which gives a link to it and where the emphasis on consumers as clients is even more noticeable (but it is impossible to tell which wording there actually comes from the OMH document). Patients in the United States *cannot but* be consumers, unlike those in, say, Canada and Sweden, where the state is the provider, not corporations.

15. A number of so-called hemorrhagic fevers exist. All of the virus families can cause hemorrhagic fevers, but they share a very limited set of common characteristics: a basic structure consisting of a core of ribonucleic acid (RNA) as the genetic material, surrounded by a fatty material; dependency on a nonhuman animal or insect host for survival; and spread to humans from the infected host; as well as (in many of them) person-to-person infection. Outbreaks may be unpredictable but do not occur outside of the areas of inhabitation of the reservoir host. In the case of Ebola, it is not yet proved but is believed that African fruit bats are the reservoir species. In the 2014 outbreak, roughly 18 percent of the infected developed hemorrhagic fever. Alan Schmaljohn, a virologist and professor of microbiology and immunology at the University of Maryland School of Medicine, states, "I've long disliked the lumping of 'hemorrhagic fever viruses' with one term, because they are such different viruses, with different physical and genetic characteristics, and hemorrhage is not a consistent feature of any of them" (cited in Palermo 2014). As Dr. Louis Katz says, "Ebola has that reputation.... But it's really just a small minority of people infected who bleed significantly" (cited in Schattner 2015). Platelets, the clotting factor in blood, do diminish in Ebola cases, but often not sufficiently to cause hemorrhagic bleeding.

16. See, for example, Coscarelli 2014.

3. Addiction and Its Formations under Capitalism

1. On March 28, 1979, Three Mile Island in southeastern Pennsylvania was the site of the worst commercial nuclear accident in history, releasing multiple noxious gases into the environment.

2. For an astute assessment of the implications of this history for the present, see Magoc 2014.

3. Dunoon is a large, Black informal settlement on the outskirts of Cape Town where tensions seethe. Anger and disgruntlement over lack of housing and services, minimal policing, massive overcrowding, resentment of large numbers of foreign African immigrants/migrants/illegals, disputes over taxi routes, and territorial gangs manifest themselves in violent outbreaks of arson, shootings, and xenophobic attacks.

4. One of the most infamous of Hendrik Verwoerd's quotations, from a policy speech on "Bantu" education, reads as follows: "There is no place for [the Bantu] in the European community above the level of certain forms of labour.... What is the use of teaching the Bantu child mathematics when it cannot use it in practice? That is quite absurd. Education must train people in accordance with their opportunities in life, according to the sphere in which they live" (Verwoerd 1954, 24). The speech is quoted and discussed in Clark and Worger 2004, 48–52.

5. The massacre of thirty-four striking platinum miners on August 16, 2012,

near the village of Marikana in South Africa marked the first deadly use of the South African police forces since apartheid (Bell 2016).

6. In this respect, Dian Million's warning that therapy geared at rendering a body fit for further capitalist extraction and production is toxic (2013), suggests even more pertinently that a refusal to hand oneself over to most projects of therapeutic rehabilitation is an aspect of persistence.

7. For more on the historical figure of Ambroise Paré, barber-surgeon to kings, see Hamby 1967.

8. For more on this history, see Zackie Achmat and the Treatment Action Campaign in South Africa, which he founded. *It's My Life* (Tilley 2001) is a film made of his refusal to take antiretroviral drugs to assert the right of all South Africans to government-provided ARVs.

4. Trauma "Exceptionalism" and Sexual Assault in Global Contexts

1. For example, when I worked on a project that had a protocol asking about the onset of what is coyly called "sexual debut" in adolescents in KwaZulu-Natal (KZN), the translators pointed out that sexual relationships among youth in that area do not see penetration as a marker of sexual intercourse, but a range of behaviors, including "thigh sex," or *ukusoma* in isiZulu. Mark Hunter discusses "thigh sex" as rejected in particularly urban modes of *isoka,* or masculinity status, but in rural areas *ukusoma* is more broadly not only recognized but practiced (2002). I recognize Hunter's careful distinctions between actual practices and the invention of "tradition," especially by elder men, such as chief's advisers (*izInduna*) and chiefs (*amaKosi*), but this does not mean the practice can be relegated to history. I take the warning of Hein De Vries et al. that statistics for sexual debut may include participants who see *ukusoma* counting as the onset as a further indication in this regard (2014, 1093). John Imrie et al. also note that researchers, overlooking *ukusoma* may lead to an inaccurate picture of HIV risk in men who have sex with men in rural South African communities (2013, S73).

2. For example, see Kappelman on the systemic violence expressed by the U. S. Department of Veteran Affairs in its obstruction of the claim of victim-survivors of MSA (military sexual assault) to services for PTSD, as opposed to survivors of non-MSA-related PTSD (2011). It is telling in this context that Kappelman refers to MSA rather than what he calls the "somewhat euphemistic" term "personal assault." This is because the latter erases the context of the military in sexual assault cases in which both perpetrator and victim are members of the armed forces.

3. See Bourdieu 2000, 142–43: "The agent engaged in practice knows the world . . . too well, without objectifying distance; he takes it for granted, precisely because he is caught up in it, bound up with it; he inhabits it like a garment; . . . he

feels at home in the world because the world is also in him, in the form of the habitus."

4. For work on the need to look at public health in Indigenous communities within the broader fabric of the negative, intergenerational health effects of settler colonialism, see Crawford 2014; Paradies 2016; James et al. 2014; Kirmayer 2015; Kirmayer et al. 2011.

5. For an excellent set of analyses of the refusal of such victimization, see Rifkin 2012. My thinking on this has also been informed by Armand Garnet Ruffo's depiction of interracial sexual assault in his acclaimed film *A Windigo Tale* and Robertson and Henderson's 2010 graphic novel series for adolescents on the intergenerational effects of abuse, including sexual abuse, in the residential school systems.

6. For excellent sources on transactional sex, see Hunter 2002 and Leclerc-Madlala 2004.

7. See, for example, the statement that "childhood abuse is an intergenerational problem" in Robertson and Henderson 2010 and Johnson and James 2016.

8. There is very little data on the clinical treatment of infant rape survivors—merely calls for research on the topic, especially from South Africa, where such rapes were reported in a spate, particularly from 2001 onward (see Pitcher and Bowley 2002; Dutton 2013; Bowley and Pitcher 2002; As, Millar, and Rode 2002; Abrahams and Mathews 2008; Cox et al. 2007; Booysen et al. 2008; Marchetti-Mercer 2003; Richter 2003; Meier 2002; Jewkes, Martin, and Penn-Kekana 2002). Researchers have found that, before age three, it is extremely difficult to trace events of trauma, including sexual trauma, to the later development of subjects, in part because discrete memory-making appears at roughly age three and after (Colarusso 2010, 8; Gaensbauer and Bauer 2009). Gaensbauer summarizes the situation thus: "Young children's cognitive immaturity does not preclude them from developing some kind of memory for a traumatic event, though children younger than 18 months of age will tend to have fewer symptoms in the reexperiencing category compared with those in older children" (Coates and Gaensbauer 2009, 616).

9. I have had extensive conversations with Professor Steve Collings on this aspect of childhood survivors' needs. Professor Collings runs a clinic for abused children and adolescents in Durban, KZN, and teaches psychology at the University of KwaZulu-Natal. Drawing and other forms of play therapy can be very effective in treating child survivors of sexual assault, but only if the child is in a stable setting at home and the therapist builds a relation of trust between the child, the physical environment of the therapist's office, and the therapist's own person (Coates and Gaensbauer 2009). Evidence suggests, too, that how children manifest symptoms after sexual assault depends on not only the repetition of

trauma (not necessarily sexual assault trauma, repetition of trauma being the most important factor in post-sexual-assault recovery), but also the *age* at the time of the assault. Prior to twelve years of age, evidence shows that children are likely to develop symptoms of depression; after age twelve, the children are ten times more likely to develop PTSD (Schoedl et al. 2010).

10. See chapter 3 of *Cultured Violence,* entitled "Women, Stigma and the Performance of Alienation," in Jolly 2010, 82–116.

11. Joseph Pierre notes the dependence of psychiatry on World War I and World War II as the precipitators or "triggers" of a preexistent predilection for mental disorder, where war itself is considered as an event, not a series of events (2013). Recognition of "battle fatigue," "combat exhaustion," and "shell-shock" among soldiers from the two wars crystallized the notion that mental illness was often precipitated by reactions to trauma, particularly among individuals with some latent "predisposition to maladjustment" (Cohen 1983, 127). Psychiatrists participated in mass screenings of prospective draftees in World War II, with 1.75 million men ultimately rejected from service based on increasing recognition of "neurotic" as opposed to "psychotic" symptoms and disorders (Horwitz 2002). These "psychoneurotic" syndromes were not catalogued within preexisting psychiatric classification manuals, necessitating revised nosologies encompassing a much broader scope of mental disorder that culminated in the publication of the first *Diagnostic and Statistical Manual of Mental Disorders* in 1952 by the Committee on Nomenclature and Statistics of the American Psychiatric Association (Pierre 2013, 107). See also Kinghorn 2013 on the history of the definition of mental disorder.

12. As Calvin Colarusso writes: "A recent study of thousands of HMO members [Anda et al. 2006] once again confirmed the relationship between early adverse childhood experiences such as childhood sexual abuse and a wide variety of psychological disorders and problems. But more importantly, the researchers also found a clear relationship between the number of adverse experiences in childhood and the degree of psychopathology in adulthood. Earlier and more intense adversity produced a greater number of maladaptive outcomes" (2010, 3).

13. This refers to the *Access Hollywood* outtake in which Donald Trump was recorded saying "When you're famous, . . . you can do anything to [women]. Grab 'em by the pussy, anything," which he subsequently defended as "locker room talk" (Victor 2017).

5. Effluent Capacity and the Human Right-Making Artifact

1. Dian Million's 2013 *Therapeutic Nations* documents the dependence of Canadian sovereignty on violence against Aboriginal women. Sarah Deer, in a

companion project, her 2015 *The Beginning and End of Rape,* articulates the intertwining of the U.S. legal system, through the Federal Indian Law, to the project of Aboriginal women's sexual victimization in the United States.

2. For histories of the terms "human" and "human right" and their definitions in the practice of the United Nations and others, see Smeulers and Grunfeld 2011. For the technical, detailed definition of "Gross Human Rights Violations" by the Human Rights Commission of the United Nations and the term's history in U.N. literature, see note 5 in the introduction.

3. Nor is it to ignore the fact that posthuman environmentalism itself often ignores: that the exploitation of world resources has been enjoyed by a privileged few and enabled by exploitative labor. Thus there is a moral question involved in asking countries on the "low" side of unequal development to be equally responsible for the (re)distribution of ecological responsibility.

4. It bears repeating that, within colonialist governance, the native's failings to conform to the norms assumed in that governance render the native "naturally" pathological. This becomes especially apparent in readings of Indigenous communities in relation to their health and sexuality. See Ahenakew 2011 for a specific contemporary example.

5. See, for example, Wright's post on the Stop the NT Intervention website, stoptheintervention.org/rda-new-legislation/comments/alexis-wright-author-4-2-10.

6. In this respect, Morton's (white) hyperobjects can be seen as "beyond settler time," to use Mark Rifkin's formulation (2017). Rifkin's work of that title explores how native concepts are forced into settler chronologies in ways that deform the very substance of those concepts.

7. I am aware of the rejections of resilience as a neoliberal tool for the governance and maintenance of the impoverished at the level of subjects and the "developing" state by Mark Neocleous (2013) and Sarah Bracke (2016). They reject it as it can be used to insist that the resilience of the poor and/or underserviced justifies the withdrawal of public-health and other services from those populations. This cannot be the case in my argument, as I am proposing that the very self-destruction of Aboriginal bodies counters their exploitation in *Carpentaria,* as the deeply ailing or dead body cannot work for the mines. For more on my choice of the term "persistence" in most contexts over "resistance" or "resilience," see the introduction.

Afterword

1. Mark Rifkin's 2017 monograph *Beyond Settler Time* deals with precisely what it means to frame Aboriginal being without invoking settler chronology.

Bibliography

Abaka, Edmund. 2007. "American Colonization Society." In *Encyclopedia of Western Colonialism Since 1450*, vol. 1, edited by Thomas Benjamin, 37–38. Macmillan Reference USA.

Abrahams, Naeemah, and Shanaaz Mathews. 2008. "Services for Child Sexual Abuse Lacking." *South African Journal of Medicine* 7 (98): 494.

Adebajo, Adekeye. 2002. *Liberia's Civil War: Nigeria, ECOMOG, and Regional Security in West Africa*. Boulder, Colo.: Lynne Rienner.

Agamben, Giorgio. 1998. *Homo Sacer: Sovereign Power and Bare Life*. Translated by Daniel Heller-Roazen. Stanford, Calif.: Stanford University Press.

Ahenakew, Cash. 2011. "The Birth of the 'Windigo': The Construction of Aboriginal Health in Biomedical and Traditional Indigenous Medicine." *Critical Literacy: Theories and Practices* 5 (1): 14–26.

Altman, John, and Susie Russel. 2012. "Too Much 'Dreaming': Evaluations of the Northern Territory National Emergency Response Intervention, 2007–2012." *Evidence Base* 3: 1–24.

American Psychiatric Association, Committee on Nomenclature and Statistics. 1952. *Diagnostic and Statistical Manual: Mental Disorders*. Washington, D.C.: American Psychiatric Association.

Anda, R. F., V. J. Felitti, J. D. Bremner, et al. 2006. "The Enduring Effects of Abuse and Related Adverse Experiences in Childhood." *European Archives of Psychiatry and Clinical Neuroscience* 256 (3): 174–86.

Anderson, Patricia, and Rex Wild. 2007. *Ampe Alkelyernemane Meke Mekarle: Little Children Are Sacred*. Report of the Board of Inquiry into the Protection of Aboriginal Children from Sexual Abuse. Darwin: Northern Territory of Australia Government.

Anderson, Warwick. 1998. "Where Is the Postcolonial History of Medicine?" *Bulletin of the History of Medicine* 72 (2): 522–30.

Andersson, Neil. 2006. "Prevention for Those Who Have Freedom of Choice—or Among the Choice-Disabled: Confronting Equity in the AIDS Epidemic." *AIDS Research and Therapy* 3: 1–3.

Anzaldúa, Gloria E. 1987. *Borderlands / La Frontera: The New Mestiza*. San Francisco: Aunt Lute.

Arendt, Hannah. [1951] 1976. *The Origins of Totalitarianism*. New edition with added prefaces. New York: Harcourt Brace Jovanovich.

Arrighi, Giovanni. 1994. *The Long Twentieth Century: Money, Power and the Origins of Our Times*. London: Verso.

As, A. B., van, A. J. W. Millar, and H. Rode. 2002. "The Rape of Infants in South Africa." *South African Medical Journal* 92 (3): 9–10.

Attridge, Derek, and Rosemary J. Jolly, eds. 1998. *Writing South Africa: Literature, Apartheid, and Democracy, 1970–1995*. Cambridge: Cambridge University Press.

Attwell, David. 1998. "'Dialogue' and 'Fulfilment' in J. M. Coetzee's *Age of Iron*." In Attridge and Jolly, *Writing South Africa*, 166–79.

Australian Human Rights Commission. 2011. *The Suspension and Reinstatement of the RDA and Special Measures in the NTER*. Sydney: Australian Human Rights Commission.

Barad, Karen. 2003. "Posthumanist Performativity: Toward an Understanding of How Matter Comes to Matter." *Signs: Journal of Women in Culture and Society* 28 (3): 801–31.

Baskas, Harriet. 2014. "Instead of Wearing an Ebola Costume, Donate One, New Campaign Says." *Today*, October 31. Accessed January 1, 2021. today.com/money/controversial-sexy-ebola-halloween-costume-sparks-donations-1d80258281.

Beckman, Ericka. 2012. "An Oil Well Named Macondo: Latin American Literature in the Time of Global Capital." *Publications of the Modern Language Association* 127 (1): 145–51.

Bell, Terry. 2016. "The Marikana Massacre: Why Heads Must Roll." *New Solutions: A Journal of Environmental and Occupational Health Policy* 25 (4): 440–50.

Benveniste, Emile. 1971. *Problems in General Linguistics*. Translated by Elizabeth Meek. Coral Gables, Fla.: University of Miami Press.

Berlant, Lauren. 2001. "The Subject of True Feeling: Pain, Privacy, Politics." In *Cultural Pluralism, Identity Politics, and the Law*, edited by Austin Sarat and Robert J. Kearns, 49–84. Ann Arbor: University of Michigan Press.

Berlant, Lauren. 2011. *Cruel Optimism*. Durham, N.C.: Duke University Press.

Bilby, Kenneth M. 2005. *True-Born Maroons*. Gainesville: University of Florida Press.

Billings, Peter. 2009. "Still Paying the Price for Benign Interventions? Contextualizing Contemporary Interventions in the Lives of Aboriginal Peoples." *Melbourne University Law Review* 33 (1): 1–38.

Bleakley, Alan, Julie Brice Brown, and John Bligh. 2008. "Thinking the Postcolonial in Medical Education." *Medical Education* 42 (3): 266–70.

Boal, Augusto. 1979. *Theater of the Oppressed*. Translated by Charles A. McBride and Odilia Neal McBride. New York: Theater Communications Group.

Boluk, Stephanie, and Wylie Lenz. 2011. "Generation Z, the Age of the Apocalypse."

In *Generation Zombie: Essays on the Living Dead in Modern Culture,* edited by Stephanie Boluk and Wylie Lenz, 1–17. Jefferson, N.C.: McFarland.
Booysen, N., C. Bown, N. Collison, et al. 2008. "The Child Rape Epidemic." *South African Journal of Medicine* 98 (7): 490–91.
Bourdieu, Pierre. 2000. *Pascalian Meditations.* Translated by R. Nice. Cambridge: Polity.
Bowley, Douglas M. G., and Graeme J. Pitcher. 2002. "Motivation behind Infant Rape in South Africa." *The Lancet* 359 (9314): 1352.
Bracke, Sarah. 2016. "Bouncing Back: Vulnerability and Resistance in Times of Resilience." In Butler, Gambetti, and Sabsay, *Vulnerability in Resistance,* 52–75.
Burin, Eric. 2005. *Slavery and the Peculiar Solution: A History of the American Colonization Society.* Gainesville: University of Florida Press.
Butler, Judith. 1997. *Excitable Speech: A Politics of the Performative.* Abingdon, UK: Routledge.
Butler, Judith. 2006. *Precarious Life: The Powers of Violence and Mourning.* London: Verso.
Butler, Judith. 2009. *Frames of War: When Is Life Grievable?* London: Verso.
Butler, Judith. 2016. "Rethinking Vulnerability and Resistance." In Butler, Gambetti, and Sabsay, *Vulnerability in Resistance,* 12–27.
Butler, Judith, Zeynep Gambetti, and Leticia Sabsay, eds. 2016. *Vulnerability in Resistance: Towards a Feminist Theory of Resistance and Agency.* Durham, N.C.: Duke University Press.
Caiola, Sammy. 2014. "Hazmat Suits Are Hot Halloween Item: Ebola Hikes Demand for Protective Gear." *The Sacramento Bee,* Our Region, 1B, October 27. Accessed January 1, 2020. sacbee.com/news/local/health-and-medicine/healthy-choices/article3391186.html.
Campbell, Mavis. 1988. *The Maroons of Jamaica 1655–1796.* Lawrenceville, N.J.: Africa World.
Carastathis, Anna. 2014. "The Concept of Intersectionality in Feminist Theory." *Philosophy Compass* 9 (5): 304–14.
Cariou, Warren. 2018. "Sweetgrass Stories: Listening for Animate Land." *Cambridge Journal of Postcolonial Inquiry* 5 (3): 338–52.
Caruth, Cathy, ed. 1995. *Trauma: Explorations in Memory.* Baltimore, Md.: Johns Hopkins University Press.
Caruth, Cathy. 1996. *Unclaimed Experience.* Baltimore, Md.: Johns Hopkins University Press.
Centers for Disease Control, National Center for HIV, Viral Hepatitis, STD, and TB Prevention. 2010. *Establishing a Holistic Framework to Reduce Inequities in HIV, Viral Hepatitis, STDs, and Tuberculosis in the United States.* White paper. March 21. Accessed September 20, 2022. cdc.gov/nchhstp/socialdeterminants/docs/SDH-White-Paper-2010.pdf.

Chari, Sharad. 2013. "Detritus in Durban: Polluted Environs and the Biopolitics of Refusal." In *Imperial Debris: On Ruins and Ruination*, edited by Laura Ann Stoler, 131–61. Durham, N.C.: Duke University Press.

Christopher, Emma. 2008. "A 'Disgrace to the Very Colour': Perceptions of Blackness and Whiteness in the founding of Sierra Leone and Botany Bay." *Journal of Colonialism and Colonial History* 9 (3).

Clark, Nancy L., and William H. Worger. 2004. *South Africa: The Rise and Fall of Apartheid*. Harlow, U.K.: Pearson Longman.

Coates, Susan, and Theodore J. Gaensbauer. 2009. "Event Trauma in Early Childhood: Symptoms, Assessment, Intervention." *Child and Adolescent Psychiatric Clinics of North America* 3 (18): 611–26.

Cock, Joan. 2012. "The Violence of Structures and the Violence of Foundings." *New Policial Science* 34 (2): 221–27.

Coetzee, J. M. 1980. *Waiting for the Barbarians*. London: Secker and Warburg.

Coetzee, J. M. 1982. "Idleness in South Africa." *Social Dynamics* 8 (1): 1–13.

Coetzee, J. M. 2007. *Diary of a Bad Year*. London: Harvill Secker.

Cohen, S. 1983. "The Mental Hygiene Movement, the Development of Personality and the School: The Medicalization of American Education." *History of Education Quarterly* 23 (2): 123–49.

Colarusso, Calvin. 2010. *The Long Shadow of Sexual Abuse: Developmental Effects across the Life Cycle*. Lanham, Md.: Jason Aronson.

Comins, Lyse. 2015. "Durban's Plan to Recycle Graves." *IOL*, September 14. Accessed February 17, 2017. iol.co.za/news/south-africa/kwazulu-natal/durbans-plan-to-recycle-graves-1915860.

Coscarelli, Joe. 2014. "Here's What Survivalists Are Buying to Prepare for the Ebola Outbreak." *New York Magazine*, October 3. Accessed January 16, 2018. nymag.com/daily/intelligencer/2014/10/how-preppers-are-stocking-up-for-ebola-outbreak.html.

Cox, S., G. Andrade, D. Lungelow, et al. 2007. "The Child Rape Epidemic: Assessing the Incidence at Red Cross Hospital, Cape Town, and Establishing the Need for a New National Protocol." *South African Journal of Medicine* 97 (10): 950–55.

Craps, Stef. 2013. *Postcolonial Witnessing: Trauma out of Bounds*. New York: Palgrave Macmillan.

Cravioto, Alejando, Claudio F. Lanata, Daniele S. Lantagne, and Balakrish G. Nair. 2011. "Final Report of the Independent Panel of Experts on the Cholera Outbreak in Haiti." United Nations, May 4. Accessed October 13, 2017. reliefweb.int/attachments/97a78ba5-990e-3627-9a6e-96a83b2e2bba/Full_Report.pdf.

Crawford, Allison. 2014. "'The Trauma Experienced by Generations Past Having an Effect in Their Descendants': Narrative Historical Trauma among the Inuit in Nunavut, Canada." *Transcultural Psychiatry* 51 (3): 339–69.

Crenshaw, Kimberle. 1991. "Mapping the Margins: Intersectionality, Identity Politics, and Violence against Women of Color." *Stanford Law Review* 43 (6): 1241–99.

Culhane, Dara. 2015. Dian Million, "Therapeutic Nations: Healing in an Age of Indigenous Human Rights." *Peace Studies: A Journal of Social Justice* 27 (3): 399–401.

Dangarembga, Tsitsi. 1989. *Nervous Conditions*. New York: Seal.

De Vries, Hein, Sander Matthijs Eggers, Champak Jinabhai, et al. 2014. "Adolescents' Beliefs about Forced Sex in KwaZulu-Natal, South Africa." *Archives of Sexual Behavior* 43: 1087–95.

Debut, Béatrice. 2015. "South Africa's New Human Ancestor Sparks Racial Row." Phys Org, September 17. Accessed August 13, 2020. phys.org/news/2015-09-south-africa-human-ancestor-racial.html.

Deer, Sarah. 2015. *The Beginning and End of Rape: Confronting Sexual Violence in Native America*. Minneapolis: University of Minnesota Press.

Diamond, Arthur. 1989. *Paul Cuffe*. New York: Chelsea House.

Douglas, Paul H. 1927. "Political History of the Occupation." In *Occupied Haiti: Being the Report of a Committee of Six Disinterested Americans Representing Organizations Exclusively American, Who, Having Personally Studied Conditions in Haiti in 1926, Favor the Restoration of the Independence of the Negro Republic,* edited by Emily Greene Balch. New York: Writers, 15–36. Accessed October 12, 2017. babel.hathitrust.org/cgi/pt?id=txu.059173022960792&view=1up&seq=31.

Dunn-Marcos, Robin, Konia T. Kollehlon, Bernard Ngovo, and Emily Russ. 2005. *Liberians: An Introduction to their History and Culture*. Edited by Donald A. Renard. Culture Profile 19. Washington, D.C.: Center for Applied Linguistics. culturalorientation.net/content/download/1358/7913/version/2/file/Liberians.pdf.

Dutton, Jessica. 2013. "Layers of Violence: A Gender Perspective on Media Reporting on Infant Rape in South Africa." In *Gendered Perspectives on Conflict and Violence : Part A,* by Marcia Texler Segal and Vasilikie P. Demos, 243–72. Bingley, U.K.: Emerald Group.

Environmental Protection Agency. 2017. "Lead Laws and Regulations." EPA: Lead, May 8. Accessed November 21, 2017. epa.gov/lead/lead-regulations#paint.

Esposito, Roberto. 2008. *Bios: Biopolitics and Philosophy*. Translated by Timothy Campbell. Minneapolis: University of Minnesota Press.

Esposito, Roberto. 2010. *Communitas: The Origin and Destiny of Community*. Translated by Timothy Campbell. Stanford, Calif.: Stanford University Press.

Esposito, Roberto. 2011. *Immunitas: The Protection and Negation of Life*. Translated by Zakiya Hanafi. Cambridge: Polity.

Esposito, Roberto. 2013. "Community, Immunity, Biopolitics." Translated by Zakiya Hanafi. *Angelaki* 18 (3): 83–90.

Eubanks, Charlotte. 2019. *The Art of Persistence: Akamatsu Toshiko and the Visual Cultures of Transwar Japan*. Honolulu: University of Hawai'i Press.

Fanon, Frantz. 1991a. *Black Skin, White Masks*. Edited and translated by C. L. Markmann. New York: Grove.

Fanon, Frantz. 1991b. *The Wretched of the Earth*. Edited and translated by C. L. Markmann. New York: Grove.

Faria, Nuno, et al. 2014. "The Early Spread and Epidemic Ignition of HIV-1 in Human Populations." *Science* 346 (6205): 56–61.

Farmer, Paul. 1992, 2006. *AIDS and Accusation: Haiti and the Geography of Blame*. Berkeley and Los Angeles: University of California Press.

Farmer, Paul. 2011. *Haiti after the Earthquake*. New York: Public Affairs.

Fortin, Jeffrey. 2006. "'Blackened beyond our Native Hue': Removal, Identity and the Trelawney Maroons on the Margins of the Atlantic World, 1796–1800." In "Freedom on the Margins." Special issue, *Citizenship Studies* 10 (1): 5–34.

Foucault, Michel. 2008. *The Birth of Biopolitics: Lectures at the College de France, 1978–1979*. Translated by G. Burchell and edited by A. I. Davidson. New York: Palgrave Macmillan.

Fyfe, Christopher. 1962. *History of Sierra Leone*. London: Oxford University Press.

Gaensbauer, Theodore J., and Leslie Bauer. 2009. "Psychoanalytic Perspectives on Early Trauma: Interviews with Thirty Analysts Who Treated an Adult Victim of a Circumscribed Trauma in Early Childhood." *Journal of the American Psychoanalytic Association* 57 (4): 947–77.

Galtung, Johan. 1969. "Violence, Peace, and Peace Research." *Journal of Peace Research* 6 (3): 167–91.

Garuba, Harry. 2003. "Explorations in Animist Materialism: Notes on Reading/Writing African Literature, Culture, and Society." *Public Culture* 15 (2): 261–86.

Giroux, Henry A. "Violence, Katrina, and the Biopolitics of Disposability." *Theory, Culture & Society* 24: 7–8.

Glissant, Éduoard. 1989. *Caribbean Discourse: Selected Essays*. Translated by Michael Dash. Charlottesville: University Press of Virginia.

Grant, John N. 2002. *The Maroons in Nova Scotia*. Halifax: Formac.

Gregory, Derek. 2004. *The Colonial Present: Afghanistan, Palestine, Iraq*. Oxford: Blackwell.

Gugelberger, Georg M. 1985. *Marxism and African Literature*. Trenton, N.J.: Africa World.

Gunne, Sorcha, and Neil Lazarus. 2012. "Mind the Gap: An Interview with Neil Lazarus." *Postcolonial Text* 7 (3): 1–15.

Haigh, Jennifer. 2016. *Heat and Light*. New York: HarperCollins.

Hamby, Wallace B. 1967. *Ambroise Paré: Surgeon of the Renaissance.* St. Louis, Mo.: Warren H. Green.

Hananoki, Eric. 2014. "Fox Doc's Racial Rant: Obama Welcomes Ebola Because His 'Affinities' Are with Africa." Media Matters, October 15. Accessed March 31, 2016. mediamatters.org/fox-news/fox-docs-racial-rant-obama-welcomes-ebola-because-his-affinities-are-africa.

Hanlon, Peter, S. Carlisle, M. Hannah, et al. 2011. "Making the Case for a 'Fifth Wave' in Public Health." *Public Health* 125 (1): 30–36.

Haraway, Donna. 2003. *The Companion Species Manifesto: Dogs, Humans, and Significant Otherness.* Chicago: Prickly Paradigm.

Harris, Wilson. 1973. *The Whole Armour and the Secret Ladder.* London: Faber.

Harvey, David. 2000. *Spaces of Hope.* Oakland: California University Press.

Harvey, David. 2011. *The Enigma of Capital and the Crises of Capitalism.* Oxford: Oxford University Press.

Hegel, G. W. F. [1807] 1977. *Phenomenology of Spirit.* Translated by A. V. Miller, with analysis and foreword by J. N. Findlay. Oxford: Oxford University Press.

Hofstadter, Richard. 1964. "The Paranoid Style in American Politics." *Harper's Magazine,* November, 77–86. harpers.org/archive/1964/11/the-paranoid-style-in-american-politics/.

Horwitz, Allan V. 2002. *Creating Mental Illness.* Chicago: University of Chicago Press.

Huber, Matthew T. 2014. "Refined Politics: Petroleum Products, Neoliberalism and the Ecology of Entrepreneurial Life." In *Oil Culture,* edited by R. Barrett and D. Worden, 226–43. Minneapolis: University of Minnesota Press.

Hund, Wulf D., and Charles W. Mills. 2016. "Comparing Black People to Monkeys Has a Long, Dark Simian History." *The Conversation,* February 28. Accessed August 13, 2020. theconversation.com/comparing-black-people-to-monkeys-has-a-long-dark-simian-history-55102.

Hunter, Mark. 2002. "The Materiality of Everyday Sex: Thinking beyond 'Prostitution.'" *African Studies* 61 (1): 99–120.

Imrie, John, Graeme Hoddinott, Sebastian Fuller, et al. 2013. "Why MSM in Rural South African Communities Should Be an HIV Prevention Research Priority." *AIDS and Behaviour* 17 (S1): S70–S76.

Ince, Onur Ulas. 2018. *Colonial Capitalism and the Dilemmas of Liberalism.* New York: Oxford University Press.

Jackson, Zakiyyah Iman. 2013. "Animal: New Directions in the Theorization of Race and Posthumanism." *Feminist Studies* 39 (3): 669–85.

James, A., K. Hopper, M. Rasmus, et al. 2014. "Mapping Resilience Pathways of Indigenous Youth in Five Circumpolar Communities." *Transcultural Psychiatry* 51 (5): 601–39.

Jewkes, Rachel, Lorna Martin, and Loveday Penn-Kekana. 2002. "The Virgin-Cleansing Myth: Cases of Child Rape Are Not Exotic." *The Lancet* 359 (9307): 711.

Johnson, Emmanuel Janagan, and Christine James. 2016. "Effects of Child Abuse and Neglect on Adult Survivors." *Early Child Development and Care* 186 (11): 1836–45.

Jolly, Rosemary J. 2010. *Cultured Violence: Narrative, Social Suffering and Engendering Human Rights in Contemporary South Africa*. Liverpool: Liverpool University Press.

Jolly, Rosemary J. 2016. "Fictions of the Human Right to Health: Writing against the Postcolonial Exotic in Western Medicine." In *The Edinburgh Companion to the Critical Medical Humanities*, edited by Anne Whitehead and Angela Woods. 527–40. Edinburgh: Edinburgh University Press.

Jolly, Rosemary J. 2020. "Pandemic Crises: The Anthropocene as Pathogenic Cycle." *Interdisciplinary Studies in Literature and Environment* 27 (4): 809–22. doi.org/10.1093/isle/isaa180.

Jolly, Rosemary J. 2022. "Decolonising 'Man,' Resituating Pandemic: An Intervention in the Pathogenesis of Colonial Capitalism." *British Medical Journal: Medical Humanities* 48 (2): 221–29.

Jolly, Rosemary J., and Alexander Fyfe. 2018. "Introduction: Reflections on Postcolonial Animations of the Material." *Cambridge Journal of Postcolonial Literary Inquiry* 5 (3): 296–303.

Jolly, Rosemary J., and Alan Jeeves. 2010. "'Yes, There Are Rights but Sometimes They Don't Work . . .': Gender Equity, HIV/AIDS, and Democracy in Rural South Africa since 1994." *Canadian Journal of African Studies* 44 (3): 524–51.

Joseph, Mario, and Brian Concannon. 2015. "European Parliament to Hear Arguments for Restitution of Haiti's Independence Debt." *Haiti Liberte*, June, 21–27. Accessed October 11, 2017. haiti-liberte.com/archives/volume6-43/European%20Parliament.asp.

Kappelman, Ben Desmond. 2011. "When Rape Isn't like Combat: The Disparity between Benefits for Post-Traumatic Stress Disorder for Combat Veterans and Benefits for Victims of Military Sexual Assault." *Suffolk University Law Review* 44 (2): 545–65.

Karimi, Faith, and Catherine E. Shoichet. 2014. "Thomas Eric Duncan: 7 Ways His Ebola Case Differs from Others in U.S." CNN, Health, October 10. Accessed October 22, 2017. cnn.com/2014/10/09/health/ebola-duncan-death-cause/index.html.

Kim, Clare Jean. 2015. *Dangerous Crossings: Race, Species, and Nature in a Multicultural Age*. Cambridge: Cambridge University Press.

Kimmerer, Robin Wall. 2014. *Braiding Sweetgrass: Indigenous Wisdom, Scientific Knowledge, and the Teachings of Plants*. Minneapolis, Minn.: Milkweed.

Kinghorn, Warren. 2013. "The Biopolitics of Defining 'Mental Disorder.'" In *Making the DSM-5*, edited by J. Paris and J. Phillips, 47–61. New York: Springer.

Kirmayer, Lawrence J. 2015. "The Health and Well-Being of Indigenous Youth." *Acta Paediatrica* 104 (1): 2–4.

Kirmayer, Lawrence J., S. Dandenau, E. Marshall, et al. 2011. "Rethinking Resilience from Indigenous Perspectives." *Canadian Journal of Psychiatry* (56): 84–91.

Klonaris, Helen. 2011. "*Zong!* The Transformation of Language into Sacred Space." SX Salon, February. Accessed August 27, 2022. smallaxe.net/sxsalon/reviews/zong-transformation-language-sacred-space.

Knight, Peter, ed. 2002. *Conspiracy Nation: The Politics of Paranoia*. New York: New York University Press.

Krog, Antjie. 1998. *Country of My Skull*. New York: Random House.

Kuykendall, R. 1993. "Hegel and Africa: An Evaluation of the Treatment of Africa in *The Philosophy of History*." *Journal of Black Studies* 23 (4): 571–81.

LaCapra, Dominick. 1994. *Representing the Holocaust: History, Theory, Trauma*. Ithaca, N.Y.: Cornell University Press.

LaCapra, Dominick. 2004. *History in Transit: Experience, Identity, Critical Theory*. Ithaca, N.Y.: Cornell University Press.

LaCapra, Dominick. 2014. *Writing History, Writing Trauma*. New ed. Baltimore, Md.: Johns Hopkins University Press.

LaCapra, Dominick. 2016. "Trauma, History, Identity: What Remains?" *History and Theory* 55 (3): 375–400.

Lamont, D. Thomas. 1988. *Paul Cuffe: Black Entrepreneur and Pan Africanist*. Urbana: University of Illinois Press.

Land, Isaac, and Andrew M. Schocket. 2008. "New Approaches to the Founding of the Sierra Leone Colony, 1786–1808." *Journal of Colonialism and Colonial History* 9 (3). Accessed October 11, 2017.

Lauro, Sarah Juliet. 2011a. "The Eco-Zombie-Environmental Critique in Zombie Fiction." In *Generation Zombie: Essays on the Living Dead in Modern Culture*, edited by Stephanie Boluk and Wylie Lenz, 54–66. Jefferson, N.C.: McFarland.

Lauro, Sarah Juliet. 2011b. "Playing Dead: Zombies Invade Performance Art . . . and Your Neighbourhood." In *Better Off Dead: The Evolution of the Zombie as Post-Human*, edited by Deborah Christie and Juliet Lauro, 205–30. New York: Fordham University Press.

Lauro, Sarah Juliet, and Karen Embry. 2008. "A Zombie Manifesto: The Nonhuman Condition in an Era of Advanced Capitalism." *Boundary 2* 35 (1): 85–108.

Leavis, F. R. 1948. *The Great Tradition*. London: Chatto and Windus.

Leclerc-Madlala, Suzanne. 2004. "Transactional Sex and the Pursuit of Modernity." CSSR working paper no. 68. Cape Town: University of Cape Town, Centre for Social Science Research..

Lethabo King, Tiffany. 2019. *The Black Shoals: Offshore Formations of Black and Native Studies.* Durham, N.C.: Duke University Press.

Limon, Marc, and Hillary Power. 2014. *History of the United Nations Special Procedures Mechanisms: Origins, Evolution, and Reform.* universal-rights.org/wp-content/uploads/2015/02/URG_HUNSP_28.01.2015_page_by_page.pdf.

Liu, P., J. Z. Jiang, X. F. Wan, et al. 2020. "Are Pangolins the Intermediate Host of the 2019 Novel Coronavirus (SARS-CoV-2)?" *PLOS Pathogens* 16 (5): e1008421. Accessed August 27, 2022. doi.org/10.1371/journal.ppat.1008421.

Liwanga, Roger-Claude. 2015. "The Meaning of Gross Violation of Human Rights: A Focus on International Tribunals' Decisions over the DRC Conflicts." *Denver Journal of International Law & Policy* 44 (1): article 6.

Loveman, Brian. 2010. *No Higher Law: American Foreign Policy and the Western Hemisphere since 1776.* Chapel Hill: University of North Carolina Press.

Lucàks, Georg. 1962. *The Meaning of Contemporary Realism.* London: Merlin.

Luyten, Patrick, Sidney J. Blatt, Boudewijn Van Houdenhove, and Jozef Corveleyn. 2006. "Depression Research and Treatment: Are We Skating to Where the Puck is Going to Be?" *Clinical Psychology Review* 26 (8): 985–99.

Luyten, Patrick, Sidney J. Blatt, B. Van Houdenhove, and Nicole Vliegen. 2008. "Equifinality, Multifinality, and the Rediscovery of the Importance of Early Experiences: Pathways from Early Adversity to Psychiatric and (Functional) Somatic Disorders." *Psychoanalytic Study of the Child* 63 (1): 27–60.

Macoun, Alissa. 2011. "Aboriginality and the Northern Territory Intervention." *Australian Journal of Political Science* 46 (3): 519–34.

Macrotrends. 2023. Global Comparative Data. "Global Metrics." Macrotrends. Accessed May 23, 2023. Macrotends.net/countries/topic-overview.

Magoc, Chris J. 2014. "Reflections on the Public Interpretation of Regional Environmental History in Western Pennsylvania." *The Public Historian* 36 (3): 50–69.

Marchetti-Mercer, M. C. 2003. "A Socio-psychological Perspective on the Phenomenon of Infant Rapes in South Africa." *South African Psychiatry Review* 6 (4): 6–14.

Mbembe, Achilles. 2003. "Necropolitics." Translated by Libby Meintjies. *Public Culture* 15 (1): 11–40.

Mbonambi, G. 2013. "Durban's Cemeteries Are Full." IOL, October 17. Accessed February 17, 2017. iol.co.za/news/south-africa/kwazulu-natal/durbans-cemeteries-are-full/1593355.

McKegney, Sam. 2007. *Magic Weapons: Aboriginal Writers Remaking Community after Residential School.* Manitoba: University of Manitoba Press.

Meier, Eileen. 2002. "Child Rape in South Africa." *Pediatric Nursing* 28 (5): 532–34.

Million, Dian. 2013. *Therapeutic Nations: Healing in an Age of Indigenous Human Rights.* Tuscon: University of Arizona Press.

Moreman, Christopher M. 2011. "Dharma of the Living Dead: A Buddhist Meditation on the Zombie." In *Zombies Are Us: Essays on the Humanity of the Walking Dead,* edited by Christopher M. Moreman and Cory James Rushton, 123–38. Jefferson, N.C.: McFarland.

Morphy, Frances, and Howard Morphy. 2013. "Anthropological Theory and Government Policy in Australia's Northern Territory: The Hegemony of the Mainstream." *American Anthropologist* 115 (2): 174–87.

Morton, Timothy. 2013. *Hyperobjects: Philosophy and Ecology after the End of the World.* Minneapolis: University of Minnesota Press.

Mphahlele, Es'kia. 1962. *The African Image.* New York: Frederick A. Praeger.

National Assembly of France. 1789. *The Declaration of the Rights of Man and of the Citizen.* Accessed January 1, 2021. constitutionnet.org/sites/default/files/declaration_of_the_rights_of_man_1789.pdf.

National Human Genome Research Center. n.d. *Personalized Medicine.* Accessed March 8, 2021. genome.gov/genetics-glossary/Personalized-Medicine.

Neocleous, Mark. 2013. "Resisting Resilience." *Radical Philosophy* 178: 2–7.

Nixon, Rob. 2011. *Slow Violence and the Environmentalism of the Poor.* Cambridge, Mass.: Harvard University Press.

Noble, Vanessa. 2013. *A School of Struggle: Durban's Medical School and the Education of Black Doctors in South Africa.* Pietermaritzburg, South Africa: University of KwaZulu-Natal Press.

Nolen, Stephanie. 2007. *28 Stories of AIDS.* New York: Walker.

Ntshanga, Masande. 2016. *The Reactive.* Columbus, Ohio: Two Dollar Radio.

Obee, Ruth. 1999. *Es'kia Mphahlele: Themes of Alienation and African Humanism.* Athens: Ohio University Press.

Office of the United Nations High Commission on Human Rights. 2008. *The Right to Health.* Fact Sheet no. 31. OHCHR, June 01. Accessed August 13, 2020. ohchr.org/sites/default/files/Documents/Publications/Factsheet31.pdf.

Oliver, Kelly. 2001. *Witnessing: Beyond Recognition.* Minneapolis: University of Minnesota Press.

Padwe, Jonathan. 2013. "Anthropocentrism." Oxford Bibliographies, August 26. Accessed August 14, 2020. oxfordbibliographies.com/view/document/obo-9780199830060/obo-9780199830060-0073.xml.

Palermo, Elizabeth. 2014. "Ebola vs. Haemorrhagic Fever: What's the Difference?" Live Science, October 9. Accessed October 22, 2017. livescience.com/48218-ebola-hemorrhagic-fever.html.

Paradies, Yin. 2016. "Colonization, Racism and Indigenous Health." *Journal of Population Research* 33: 83–96.

Parry, Benita. 1998. "Speech and Silence in the Fictions of J. M. Coetzee." In Attridge and Jolly, *Writing South Africa,* 149–65.

Pierre, Joseph M. 2013. "Overdiagnosis, Underdiagnosis, Synthesis: A Dialectic for

Psychiatry and the DSM." In *Making the DSM-V*, edited by J. Paris and J. Phillips, 105–24. New York: Springer.
Philip, Marlene NourbeSe. 1989. "Discourse on the Logic of Language." In *She Tries Her Tongue: Her Silence Softly Breaks*, 44–46. Charlottetown, Canada: Ragweed.
Philip, Marlene NourbeSe, and Setaey Adamu Boateng. 2008. *Zong!* Middleton, Conn.: Wesleyan University Press.
Pitcher, Graeme J., and Douglas M. G. Bowley. 2002. "Infant Rape in South Africa." *The Lancet* 359 (9303): 274–75.
Povinelli, Elizabeth. 1995. "Do Rocks Listen? The Cultural Politics of Apprehending Australian Aboriginal Labor." *American Anthropologist*, n.s., 97 (3): 505–18.
Povinelli, Elizabeth. 2006. *Empire of Love: Toward a Theory of Intimacy, Genealogy, and Carnality*. Durham, N.C.: Duke University Press.
Povinelli, Elizabeth. 2011. *Economies of Abandonment: Social Endurance and Belonging in Late Liberalism*. Durham, N.C.: Duke University Press.
Povinelli, Elizabeth. 2014. "'Native Life': Or, Being outside the Carbon Imaginary." Lecture hosted by the Institute for Science, Innovation, and Society, Oxford Martin School, Oxford, March 7.
Povinelli, Elizabeth. 2016. *Geontologies: A Requiem to Late Liberalism*. Durham, N.C.: Duke University Press.
Puar, Jasbir. 2017. *The Right to Maim: Debility, Capacity, Disability*. Durham, N.C.: Duke University Press.
Pybus, Oliver G., Andrew J. Tatem, and Phillipe Lemey. 2015. "Virus Evolution and Transmission in an Ever More Connected World." *Royal Society Proceedings: Biological Sciences* 282 (1821): 2014–78.
Ravenscroft, Alison. 2010. "Carpentaria and Its Critics." *Cultural Studies Review* 16 (2): 194–224.
Redress: Seeking Reparation for Torture Survivors. 2006. "Victims, Perpetrators or Heroes? Child Soldiers before the International Criminal Court." Redress. September. Accessed October 4, 2017. redress.org/downloads/publications/childsoldiers.pdf.
Richter, Linda M. 2003. "Baby Rape in South Africa." *Child Abuse Review* 12 (6): 392–400.
Rifkin, Mark. 2012. *The Erotics of Sovereignty: Queer Native Writing in the Era of Self-Determination*. Minneapolis: University of Minnesota Press.
Rifkin, Mark. 2017. *Beyond Settler Time: Temporal Sovereignty and Indigenous Self-Determination*. Durham, N.C.: Duke University Press.
Robertson, David Alexander, and Scott B. Henderson (illustrator). 2010. *7 Generations: A Plains Cree Saga*. Winnipeg: Highwater.
Ross, Fiona C. 2002. *Bearing Witness: Women and the Truth and Reconciliation Commission in South Africa*. London: Pluto.

Rothberg, Michael. 2009. *Multiditrectional Memory: Remembering the Holocaust in the Age of Decolonization*. Stanford, Calif.: Stanford University Press.

Ruffo, Armand Garnet, dir. *A Windigo Tale*. 2010.

Ryn, Zdzisław Jan, and Stanisław Kłodziński. 2017. "Teetering on the Brink between Life and Death: A Study on the Concentration Camp *Muselmann*." *Medical Review—Auschwitz*, August 21, 27–73. Originally published as "Na granicy życia i śmierci. Studium obozowego 'muzułmaństwa.'" *Przegląd Lekarski—Oświęcim*, 1983.

Sale, Maggie Montesinos. 1997. *The Slumbering Volcano: American Slave Ship Revolts and the Production of Rebellious Masculinity*. Durham, N.C.: Duke University Press.

Samin, Richard. 1997. "Interview: Richard Samin with Es'kia Mphahlele." *Research in African Literature* 28 (4): 182–200.

Schama, Simon. 2006. *Rough Crossings: The Slaves, the British, and the American Revolution*. New York: Ecco.

Schattner, Elaine. 2015. "Why Some Ebola Patients Bleed, and How Plasma Might Help Recovery." *Forbes*, October 14. Accessed October 22, 2017. forbes.com/sites/elaineschattner/2014/10/15/why-some-ebola-patients-bleed-and-how-plasma-might-help-recovery/#7200b8192a16.

Schmidt, Hans. 1995. *The United States Occupation of Haiti, 1915–1934*. New Brunswick, N.J.: Rutgers University Press.

Schoedl, A. Ferri, M. C. P. Costa, J. J. Mari, et al. 2010. "The Clinical Correlates of Reported Childhood Sexual Abuse: An Association between Age at Trauma Onset and Severity of Depression and PTSD in Adults." *Journal of Child Sexual Abuse* 19 (2): 156–70.

Seligman, Herbert J. 1920. "Conquest of Haiti." In *Selections from "The Nation Magazine," 1865–1990*, edited by Katerina Vanden Heuvel. New York: Thunder's Mouth, 1990. Accessed at Third World Traveler, October 13, 2017. thirdworldtraveler.com/Independent_Media/Conquest_Haiti_SNM.html.

Senauth, Frank. 2011. *The Making and the Destruction of Haiti*. Bloomington, Ind.: AuthorHouse.

Sengupta, Somini. 2016. "U.N. Apologizes for Role in Haiti's 2010 Cholera Outbreak." *New York Times*, December 1. Accessed October 13, 2017. nytimes.com/2016/12/01/world/americas/united-nations-apology-haiti-cholera.html.

Sharpe, Christina. 2016. *In the Wake: On Blackness and Being*. Durham, N.C.: Duke University Press.

Sherwood, Marika. 2007. *After Abolition: Britain and the Slave Trade since 1807*. London: IB Tauris.

Shi, Zhengli, and Zhihong Hu. 2008. "A Review of Studies on Animal Reservoirs of the SARS Coronavirus." *Virus Research* 133 (1): 74–87.

Simpson, Leanne Betasamosake. 2013. *Islands of Decolonial Love*. Winnipeg: Arbeiter Ring.

Slaughter, Joseph. 2007. *Human Rights, Inc.: The World Novel, Narrative Form, and International Law*. New York: Fordham University Press.

Smeulers, Alette, and Fred Grunfeld. 2011. *International Crimes and Other Gross Human Rights Violations: A Multi- and Interdisciplinary Textbook*. Leiden: Brill.

Solomon, Jane. 2008. *Living with X—A Body Mapping Journal in the Time of HIV and AIDS: Facilitator's Guide*. Psychosocial Wellbeing Series. Johannesburg: Regional Psychosocial Support Initiatives (REPSSI).

South Africa National Department of Health. 2012. *2011 National Antenatal Sentinel HIV and Syphilis Prevalence Survey in South Africa*. Government Report. Pretoria: National Department of Health Directorate of Epidemiology & Surveillance.

Soyinka, Wole. 1975. *Death and the King's Horseman*. New York: Norton.

Soyinka, Wole. 1976. *Myth, Literature and the African World*. Cambridge: Cambridge University Press.

Suleiman, Susan. 1990. *Subversive Intent: Gender, Politics, and the Avant-Garde*. Cambridge, Mass.: Harvard University Press.

Sutherland, Sharon, and Sarah Swan. 2011. "'Corporate Zombies' and the Perils of 'Zombie Litigation': The Walking Dead in American Judicial Writing." In *Zombies Are Us: Essays on the Humanity of the Walking Dead*, by Christopher M. Moreman and Cory James Rushton, 76–84. Jefferson, N.C.: McFarland.

Tallbear, Kim. 2015. "Theorizing Queer Inhumanisms: An Indigenous Reflection on Working beyond the Human / Not Human." *GLQ: A Journal of Lesbian and Gay Studies* 21 (2–3): 230–35.

Thomson, Rosemarie Garland. [1997] 2017. *Extraordinary Bodies: Figuring Physical Disability in American Culture and Literature*. New York: Columbia University Press.

Tilley, Brian, dir. 2001. *It's My Life*. Featuring Zackie Achmat. First Run/Icarus.

UNAIDS (Joint U.N. Programme on HIV and AIDS). 2021. *Country Factsheet: Lesotho*. United Nations. Accessed May 23, 2023. unaids.org/en/regionscountries/countries/lesotho.

United Nations. 1948. *The Universal Declaration of Human Rights*. Accessed August 27, 2022. un.org/en/about-us/universal-declaration-of-human-rights.

United Nations. 2007. *Declaration on the Rights of Indigenous Peoples*. U.N. Department of Economic and Social Affairs: Indigenous Peoples, September 13. Accessed January 1, 2021. un.org/development/desa/indigenouspeoples/wp-content/uploads/sites/19/2018/11/UNDRIP_E_web.pdf.

United Nations. 2023. *Human Development Insights*. Human Development Reports. U. N. Development Program. Accessed May 23, 2023. hdr.undp.org/data-center/country-insights#/ranks.

U.N. World Conference on Human Rights in Vienna. 1993. *Vienna Declaration and Programme of Action*. Adopted June 25. www.ohchr.org/en/instruments-mechanisms/instruments/vienna-declaration-and-programme-action.

U.S. Department of Health and Human Services, Office of Minority Health. n.d.a. OMH Rsource Center. Accessed June 12, 2023. minorityhealth.hhs.gov/omh/browse.aspx?lvl=1&lvlid=3.

U.S. Department of Health and Human Services, Office of Minority Health. n.d.b. "What Is Cultural Competency?" Office of Minority Health. Accessed October 20, 2017. Infanthearing.org/coordinator_toolkit/section10/36_cultural_competency.pdf.

Veracini, Lorenzo. 2015. *The Settler Colonial Present*. New York: Palgrave Macmillan.

Verwoerd, Hendrik Frensch. 1954. *Bantu Education: Policy for the Immediate Future*. South Africa Information Service of the Department of Native Affairs.

Victor, Daniel. 2017. "*Access Hollywood* Reminds Trump: 'The Tape Is Very Real.'" *New York Times*, November 28. Accessed January 20, 2018. nytimes.com/2017/11/28/us/politics/donald-trump-tape.html.

Vitali, Ali, Kasie Hunt, and Frank Thorp. 2018. "Trump Referred to Haiti and African Nations as 'Shithole' Countries." *NBC News*, January 11. Accessed January 1, 2021. nbcnews.com/politics/white-house/trump-referred-haiti-african-countries-shithole-nations-n836946.

Volsky, Igor. 2014. "Rush Limbaugh: Obama Wants Americans to Get Ebola as Payback for Slavery." *ThinkProgress*, October 6. Accessed October 10, 2017. thinkprogress.org/rush-limbaugh-obama-wants-americans-to-get-ebola-as-payback-for-slavery-ddf50bfc8056/.

Vorobej, Mark. 2008. "Structural Violence." *Canadian Journal of Peace and Conflict Studies* 40 (2): 84–98.

Vujnovic, Marina. 2017. "Hypercapitalism." In *The Wiley-Blackwell Encyclopedia of Globalization*. Wiley Online Library, June 22. Accessed August 14, 2020. onlinelibrary.wiley.com/doi/epdf/10.1002/9780470670590.wbeog278.pub2.

Wacquant, L. 2005. "Habitus." In *International Encyclopedia of Economic Sociology*, edited by J. Becket and Z. Milan, 317–21. London: Routledge.

Warwick Research Collective. 2015. *Combined and Uneven Development: Towards a New Theory of World-Literature*. Liverpool: Liverpool University Press.

Watt, Ian. [1957] 2001. *The Rise of the Novel: Studies in Defoe, Richardson and Fielding*. Berkley and Los Angeles: University of California Press.

Webster, Jane. 2007. "The *Zong* in the Context of the Eighteenth-Century Slave Trade." *The Journal of Legal History* 28 (3): 285–98.

Wegmann, Andrew N. 2010. "Christian Community and the Development of an Americo-Liberian Identity, 1824–1878." Master's thesis, Louisiana State University. digitalcommons.lsu.edu/gradschool_theses/525.

Weheliye, Alexander G. 2014. *Habeas Viscus: Racializing Assemblages, Biopolitics, and Black Feminist Theories of the Human.* Durham, N.C.: Duke University Press.

Wikipedia. n.d. "Liberia." *Wikipedia: Liberia.* Accessed May 23, 2023. en.wikipedia.org/wiki/Liberia#cite_note-warrant-29.

Winter, Yves. 2012. "Violence and Visibility." *New Political Science* 34 (2): 195–202.

World Health Organization. 2003. "Alert, Verification and Public Health Management of SARS in the Post-outbreak Period." Meeting Report. World Health Organization, August 14. Accessed August 14, 2020. who.int/publications/m/item/alert-verification-and-public-health-management-of-sars-in-the-post-outbreak-period.

World Health Organization. 2017a. *Global Action Plan on HIV Drug Resistance 2017–2021.* July. World Health Organization. Accessed May 23, 2023. who.int/publications/i/item/978-92-4-151284-8.

World Health Organization. 2017b. "Human Rights and Health." World Health Organization, December 29. Accessed February 5, 2020. who.int/news-room/fact-sheets/detail/human-rights-and-health.

World Health Organization, Commission on Social Determinants of Health. 2008. "Closing the Gap in a Generation: Health Equity through Action on the Social Determinants of Health." Final report of the Commission. World Health Organization, August 27. Accessed October 20, 2017. who.int/publications/i/item/WHO-IER-CSDH-08.1.

Wright, Alexis. 1997. *Grog War.* Broome, Australia: Magabala.

Wright, Alexis. 2006. *Carpentaria.* New York: Atria.

Wright, Robin. 2017. Review of *Geontologies,* by Elizabeth Povinelli. *Society + Space,* March 1. Accessed January 2020. societyandspace.org/articles/geontologies-by-elizabeth-povinelli.

Wynter, Sylvia. 2003. "Unsettling the Coloniality of Being/Power/Truth/Freedom: Towards the Human, after Man, Its Overrepresentation—An Argument." *CR: The New Centennial Review* 3 (3): 257–337.

Yeats, William Butler. 1989. *The Collected Poems of W.B. Yeats.* Edited by Richard J. Finneran. London: Palgrave Macmillan.

York, Geoffrey. 2010. "Canadian Doctors Fear 'Life and Death' Crisis at African AIDS Clinic." *Globe and Mail,* March 11. Accessed October 21, 2017. theglobeandmail.com/news/world/canadian-doctors-fear-life-and-death-crisis-at-african-aids-clinic/article4352233/.

Index

Ablow, Keith, 52–53, 55
Aboriginal peoples, 159, 189, 190; bodies of, 167, 169, 204n7; culture of, 144, 169, 177, 180; excluded from the UNDHR, 160, 161; human rights claims, 160, 162–63, 174–75, 177, 181–82, 185; labor of, 165, 176; living under colonial capitalism, 163, 165, 166–68, 172, 175–76, 177; perceived vulnerability of, 131, 132; settler treaties with, 129–30; sexual violence against, 124, 131, 161, 162; youth, 165–66, 169. See also Australia, treatment of Aboriginal citizens; Indigenous peoples
Achmat, Zackie, 114–15, 201n8
addiction, 118, 139, 186, 188; capitalism's relation to, 100–103, 107; extractive industries compared to, 94–121. See also self-harm; substance abuse
affirmation, 12, 39, 92–93, 97, 120, 126, 151, 153, 191
afterbirth: burial of, 36–37, 39. See also placenta
Agamben, Giorgio, 54, 74, 75, 199n13; on shame of victim-survivors, 151, 152, 153
AIDS. See HIV/AIDS
Althusser, Louis, 6
ancestors, 41, 45–46, 96, 118; relations with the unborn and the living, 35–37, 39, 57, 186, 189

Anderson, Patricia, 162, 163
Anderson, Warwick, 59–60, 61, 76
Andersson, Neil, 194–95n10
animals. See nonhuman animals
animism, 175, 196n11; African, 27, 34, 35, 195n1; definition of, 27; materialist, 36, 39
Anthropocene, the, 3–4, 22, 124
anthropocentrism, 11, 30, 32, 37, 46, 198n8; of colonial capitalism, 22, 24, 63; Enlightenment/post-Enlightenment, 28, 34, 35; of human rights, 31, 124, 164, 182; use of term, 16–17, 160
anthroponoses, 21–22
Anzaldúa, Gloria, 4
apartheid, 38, 101, 114, 136, 185, 194n5, 197n17; family separations during and after, 40, 45–46; trauma of, 136, 140, 141, 150. See also South Africa
Arendt, Hannah, 2, 17, 49, 195–96n7
Arrighi, Giovanni, 1; *The Long Twentieth Century*, 159
Attwell, David, 195n2
Australia: colonialist-capitalist governance, 168, 177, 180; treatment of Aboriginal citizens, 16, 143, 161, 163, 174–76, 185, 194n6. See also Northern Territory Emergency Intervention (NTER, Australia); Stronger Futures Act (Australia)

221

Baartman, Sarah, 12
Badiou, Alain, 95
Barad, Karen, 39, 196n9
Basotho HIV/AIDS clinic (Lesotho), 77–79
Beckman, Erica, 94–95, 99
being: co-constituted, 95; extra-anthropocentric, 23, 47, 187. *See also* effluent being; human beings
Benveniste, Emile, 94, 118
Berger, Philip, 77–78
Berlant, Lauren: on suffering, 125, 148; on trauma, 143, 144, 147. *See also* cruel optimism, Berlant's theory of
Bhabha, Homi, 125
bildungsroman, 19, 92–93; claiming human rights through, 26, 63, 90, 96, 164, 166; Slaughter on, 24, 26, 90, 93, 164. *See also* narratives; novels
Billings, Peter, 163
biopolitics, 54, 55, 63, 85, 189; of debility, 73–75, 83; of immunization, 82–83. *See also* let live, make die; politics
bios, 74; *zoe* versus, 75, 83. *See also* geos-bios divide
Black Lives Matter, 19, 91. *See also* racism
Blackness/Blacks, 4, 75, 189, 197n17; bodies of, 39, 167; exclusion of, 36, 58, 64; and HIV/AIDS epidemic, 54–55; middle class, 115, 119; seen as nonhuman objects, 17, 25, 62; in South Africa, 14, 115; as victims, 141, 190; whites' belief in their superiority to, 55, 64, 68, 69. *See also* race
Bleakley, Alan, 76
Bligh, John, 76
Boateng, Setaey Adamu, 8
bodies: Aboriginal, 167, 169, 204n7; Black, 39, 167; burial of, 40–42; capitalism's relation to, 106–7, 108, 121; colonizing, 60, 167; as effluent, 5, 7, 14, 39, 45–46, 80–81
body-mapping, 153–55
body-snatching, 11, 12, 194–95n10. *See also* slavery/slaves
Bourdieu, Pierre, 87, 129
Bracke, Sarah, 195n4, 204n7
Browne, Julie Brice, 76
Bruce, Susan, 95
bubble, the, 88–93, 98, 115; as containment, 94, 125–26, 136, 190; in *Heat and Light*, 93, 101–2, 108, 120–21; in *The Reactive*, 108
burials: of afterbirth, 36–37, 39; during HIV/AIDS epidemic, 40–42
Butler, Judith, 100, 113, 151, 195n3, 196n12. *See also* disposability, Butler's concept of; grievability, Butler's concept of; precarity, Butler's concept of; speakability, Butler's concept of; ungrievability, Butler's concept of; unspeakability, Butler's concept of

Canada: American Revolution Black Loyalists settled in, 65, 66; healthcare system in, 88; Indigenous peoples in, 16, 130; medical students from, 77
capitalism, 15, 17, 29, 31, 38, 110, 119, 172, 195n5; addiction's relation to, 100–103, 107; biomedical regimes under, 83; body's relation to, 106–7, 108, 121; boom-bust cycles, 119; fiction of, 94, 95, 99; interdependency rendered by, 32–33; nexus with whiteness and colonialism, 171; subvention demands, 26, 167; U.S., 95, 100. *See also* colonial capitalism; global capitalism; late capitalism;

settler capitalism; settler-colonial capitalism
Cariou, Warren, "Sweetgrass Stories: Listening for Animate Land," 38
Carpentaria Peninsula (Australia), 18. *See also* Waanyi; Wright, Alexis, *Carpentaria*; Yarralin *manngyin*
Cartesianism, 27, 38–39, 173, 188, 191, 196n9
Caruth, Cathy, 143
Castoriadis, Cornelius, 95
Centocow mission (KwaZulu-Natal, South Africa), 42–44. *See also* Stankiewicz, Ignatius
Centocow region (KwaZulu-Natal, South Africa), 14, 45–46
Chakrabarty, Dipesh, 99
child rape, 133–34. *See also* infant rape
children: exposure to lead, 89; perceived vulnerability of, 131, 132; protecting from slavery, 167; sexual assault of, 126–27, 132–38, 140, 145, 161–63, 202n8, 202–3n9, 203n12
choice disabled, 194–95n10
cholera, 72–73, 136, 199n12
citizens/citizenship, 35, 45, 54, 57–58; obtaining rights through, 50, 195–96n7; protection of, 146–47
citizen-subjects, 2–3, 50, 83–84, 185. *See also* subjects
Cock, Joan, 129–30
Coetzee, J. M.: *Diary of a Bad Year*, 40; *Foe*, 195n2; *Waiting for the Barbarians*, 183–86
coffin flies, 197n19
Colarusso, Calvin, 203n12
Collings, Steve, 202–3n9
colonial capitalism, 35, 66, 81, 83, 88, 98, 118, 184, 190; Aboriginal peoples living under, 163, 165, 166–68, 172, 175–76, 177; anthropocentric, 22, 24, 63; biopolitics and, 73–75; and causes of Ebola and HIV, 52–60; culture of, 22, 114, 171; dependence on exploited workers and slave labor, 51, 57, 68, 74, 75, 84; development of, 89–90, 124; economy of, 120, 168; effluent threatened by, 13, 14; fifth-wave public-health theory and, 166–69; governance regimes of, 125, 159, 168, 181, 204n4; harm reduction response to, 14–15, 159, 166–69, 181; human rights under, 4, 92–93; legacies of, 85; management practices, 67; otherness and, 74, 75, 90–91, 188; polarities required, 123; racist governance intersecting with, 57, 189; relations of, 11–12; resilience of, 27; resistance to, 167; sovereignty of, 84; the state and, 57, 91–92, 188; structural violence of, 51, 58, 63, 86, 115, 166, 191; subjects of, 26, 64, 74; substance abuse and, 87–121; use of term, 1, 159; values of, 86, 129; violence of, 94, 112, 198n7. *See also* capitalism; global capitalism; late capitalism; settler capitalism; settler-colonial capitalism
colonialism, 3, 25, 29, 51, 79, 144, 159, 162; commodification of, 148–49; health's relation to, 50–51, 57, 58; history of, 1, 30; nexus with whiteness and capitalism, 171. *See also* decolonialism; neocolonialism; power, colonial; settler-colonial capitalism; settler colonialism
colonization, 29, 60, 123, 149, 180; focus on humanities, 165–66; trauma of, 141, 191; whites' practices of, 3, 94, 171. *See also* decolonization
combined and unequal development, WReC's theory of, 89–90, 95

commodification/commodities, 12, 66, 84, 144, 146–49, 171
communities. *See* effluent communities; postcolonialism, communities under
Covid-19, 20–22, 51, 55, 56, 58, 188
Craps, Stef, 138, 140
Crenshaw, Kimberle, 128, 129
cruel optimism: Berlant's theory of, 98, 113–17, 120, 143, 149, 168, 169
Culhane, Dara, 191
cultural competence, 76–77; definition of, 199n14
cultural despair: use of term, 130
culture, 34, 76, 130, 144, 194n7; Aboriginal, 144, 169, 177, 180; colonialist-capitalist, 22, 114, 171; of confession, 104–5; definition of, 199n14; of effluence, 196n9; Enlightenment, 34; isiZulu, 41; settler, 156–57, 174; Western, 189

Dangarembga, Tsitsi, *Nervous Conditions,* 95–96, 110, 166
deaths, 23–24, 74, 80, 118; during HIV/AIDS epidemic, 40–46, 50. *See also* necropolitics; slow death; thanatopolitics
debility, 59, 84; in postcolonial state, 50–51, 73–75, 85
decolonialism, 4, 19, 38, 113, 161, 166, 188; in *Carpentaria,* 157; history of medicine in relation to, 19, 51, 61–62; politics of, 166; social history of, 60, 111. *See also* colonialism
decolonization, 1–4, 147, 161, 189. *See also* colonization
Defoe, Daniel, 89–90; *Robinson Crusoe,* 26
democracy, 1, 70, 130, 131, 134
development. *See* combined and uneven development, WReC's theory of
De Vries, Hein, 201n1
discrimination. *See* racism
disease(s), 57, 187–88; anthroponotic, 22; effluence in, 49–86; Haiti associated with, 70; suffering caused by, 53, 187; zoonotic, 22. *See also* health/health care; medicine; pandemics; *and individual diseases*
disposability, 75; Butler's concept of, 12, 29, 147; inadequacy to the effluent, 29–47
Doctors of the World, 52
Douglas, Paul H., 70
Duncan, Thomas Eric, 81

Eagleton, Terry, 99
Ebola, 51–62, 80, 81, 82, 85, 200n15. *See also* Halloween, Ebola costumes for
effluence, 39, 51, 196n9; capacity of, 159–82; culture of, 196n9; description of, 11–12; in disease, 49–86; as extra-anthropocentric conceit, 3–4; genre of, 90; health care in relation to, 13–14; human right-making and, 159–82; methodologies and epistemologies of, 17, 123–57; poetics of, 6–8; as remainder, 147–48, 152, 153
effluent being, 5, 6, 12, 46
effluent communities, 23–24, 36, 84–85; co-constituted, 83; grievability/ungrievability in, 40–47, 90, 91–92; narratives of, 28, 32; persistence in, 86, 93, 153; resilience within, 33, 112–21, 124; survival of, 104
effluent eye, 4–15, 23, 50–51, 57, 82
effluent subjects, 33–35, 39, 56–58, 61, 83–84; in *Heat and Light,* 102; rights of, 28, 45–46. *See also* subjectivities, effluent; subjects

embodiment, 11, 22, 25, 36–37, 113, 187, 198n2
England, Katherine, 178
English (language), 23, 27, 35, 36, 39, 197n17
Enlightenment, 28, 34, 37, 62. *See also* post-Enlightenment
environment/environmentalism, 3, 11; posthuman, 1, 204n3; subjectivities of, 6, 174; use of term, 193n3
Esposito, Roberto: on immunity, 82–83, 85, 112–13
Europe/Europeans, 37, 60, 68, 114, 136, 143, 200n4; European Man, 17, 28; Western, 3, 84, 89
extractive industries: addiction compared to, 94–121; economy of, 98–99, 102–3; exploitative practices, 19, 94, 204n3; sexual assault compared to, 124; in South Africa, 100–101. *See also* fracking

Fanon, Frantz, 17, 25, 60
Farmer, Paul, 198n7
fetish/fetishism, 11–12, 22, 29, 143, 177, 188, 197n17; definitions of, 54, 181
fifth-wave public-health theory, 18, 136, 166–69, 188. *See also* health/health care; public health
Fisher, Mark, 95
forum theater, 153–55
Foucault, Michel, 6, 33, 54, 74, 75, 83, 84
fracking, 15, 94, 98–99, 102–3, 106, 124. *See also* extractive industries
Freud, Sigmund, 25
fugue, 11; definition of, 8–9
Fyfe, Christopher, 65, 195n1

Gaensbauer, Theodore J., 202n8
Galtung, Johan, 128–29, 198n7
Gambetti, Zeynep, 195n3

Garuba, Harry, 36, 39
gender-based-violence (GBV), 134–38; extractive industry compared to, 126; harm-reduction strategy applied to, 188–91; against Indigenous women, 124; in KwaZulu-Natal, 140–41, 155; perpetrators of, 154–56, 161; victim-survivors of, 134, 155–56. *See also* rape; sexual assault
genre of man: disease in, 51, 187; normate human beings and, 126–27, 184, 186; Wynter's concept of, 3, 17, 19, 50, 124, 159–60, 186
genre of the human, 18, 27, 29, 58, 62, 187; African humanism's likeness to, 35–36; in *Carpentaria*, 166, 188; existential problem of death, 23–24; human rights invested in, 3, 47, 195n3; interdisciplinary, 24–25; normates and, 130, 191; rejection of, 4–5, 28; treatment in the UNDHR, 51, 57, 63, 160; Western, 26, 28, 34; Wynter's concept of, 17, 27, 50, 164. *See also* human beings
geobiography, 169–82, 186, 190
geos-bios divide, 176–77, 180. *See also* *bios*
Giroux, Henry, 75
Glissant, Édouard, 189
global capitalism, 1, 13, 83, 87, 110, 195n5; dependence on exploited workers and slave labor, 74; persistence under, 112–21; structural violence of, 1, 18, 61. *See also* capitalism; colonial capitalism; settler capitalism; settler-colonial capitalism
governance, 80, 182, 195n5; colonialist-capitalist, 125, 159, 168, 181, 204n4; European colonial, 136; imperial forms of, 5–6; liberal, 126–27,

129–30, 177, 179–80, 188; neoliberal, 176; racist, 57, 189; settler-colonialist, 163. *See also* nation-state; state, the
grievability, 38; Butler's concept of, 4, 33–34, 35–36, 46, 49, 127; within effluent communities, 39, 40–47, 91–92
gross human rights violations (GHRVs), 12–13; definition of, 194n5. *See also* human rights violations (HRVs)
Gugelberger, Georg M., *Marxism and African Literature*, 30

HAART. *See* highly active antiretroviral therapy (HAART)
habitus, 87, 129, 201–2n3
Haigh, Jennifer, *Heat and Light*, 85, 87–90, 94–121, 188; bubble in, 93, 101–2; *The Reactive* compared to, 87, 89–90, 186–88
Haiti: call for reparations for slavery, 69–73, 84; cholera in, 72–73; HIV/AIDS in, 70, 79–80; prejudice against, 199n11
Halloween: Ebola costumes for, 52, 54, 55–57, 58, 62–63, 80, 81. *See also* Ebola
Hanlon, Peter S., 18. *See also* fifth-wave public-health theory
Haraway, Donna, 198n6
harm reduction: applied to gender-based-violence (GBV), 188–91; mastering carbon-imaginary values, 180; as persistence, 163–66; response to colonial capitalism, 14–15, 159, 166–69, 181
Harris, Wilson, 123–24, 150; *Guyana Quartet*, 195n2

Harvey, David, 1, 84
health/health care: commodification's relation to, 50–51, 58; definition of, 119; extra-anthropocentric, 13–14; human right to, 15–22, 49–51; Indigenous peoples' obstacles to, 191; socio-political determinants of, 52, 73; state's role in, 49, 54; structural violence's effects on, 59, 85, 198n7; white colonial-settler's right to, 88. *See also* disease(s); fifth-wave public-health theory; highly active antiretroviral therapy (HAART); medicine; public health; social and economic determinants of health (SEDH); World Health Organization (WHO)
Hegel, Georg Wilhelm Friedrich, 197n18
highly active antiretroviral therapy (HAART): mapping progress of patients on, 154; medical care required while taking, 79; necessity of, 114–15; refusal to take, 14, 201n8; right to, 40, 45; state rollout of, 24, 44, 110, 118; use in Lesotho, 77
Hirsch, Marianne, 26, 27, 164
HIV/AIDS, 60, 61, 62, 197n15; deaths from, 40–46, 50; in Haiti, 70, 79–80; in Lesotho, 77–79, 80; origins of, 19–20; self-infecting, 96–97, 103, 113; testing positive for, 95, 108. *See also* highly active antiretroviral therapy (HAART); South Africa, HIV/AIDS epidemic in
Holocaust: trauma of, 4, 139–40, 141
Huber, Matthew T., 33
Huggan, Graham, 170–71
human beings, 36, 63, 159–60, 186–87; instrumentalization of, 54, 60, 172;

Western notion of, 2–3, 4. *See also* genre of the human
humanism: liberal, 24, 26, 28, 190; normate, 130; post-Enlightenment Eurocentric, 35; relation between African and European, 37; scholars of, 138–39
humanism, African, 44, 196n10; Mphahlele's concept of, 24, 34–40, 46, 161, 186, 187, 189, 196n8
humanitarianism, 3, 52, 58, 72, 80, 85–86, 138, 199n12
humanities, 4, 139, 141, 165–66
human right-making, 4–6, 23, 159–82, 185; extra-anthropocentric, 173–82
human rightness: extra-anthropocentric, 23, 31–32; nonanthropocentric, 47, 197n14
human rights, 45, 165; Aboriginal peoples' claims to, 160, 162–63, 174–75, 177, 181–82, 185; anthropocentric, 31, 124, 164, 182; bildungsroman as manifestation of, 26, 63, 90, 96, 164, 166; under colonialist-capitalist, 4, 92–93; commanding, 30; extra-anthropocentric, 5–6, 164, 169, 171, 177; in face of decolonization, 1–4; genre of, 32, 195n3; to health/health care, 15–22, 49–51; normative, 1–2, 3, 4–5, 13, 23, 24–28, 177; orthodox, 31, 46; reframing, 90, 163–66, 197n14; values of, 2–3, 17
human rights violations (HRVs), 60, 166, 194n5. *See also* gross human rights violations (GHRVs)
Hunter, Mark, 201n1
hypercapitalism, 17, 32; definition of, 194n7
hyperobjectivity/hyperobjects: Morton's concept of, 63, 169, 174, 181–82, 190, 204n4. *See also* object(s)

imaginaries: carbon, 175–78, 180; effluent, 39; Enlightenment, 62; extra-anthropocentric, 171; geo-biographical, 176; nonlinear, 189; settler-colonial, 184; settler-state, 57
immunization/immunity, 56, 64, 84; Esposito on, 82–83, 85, 112–13
imperialism, 5–6, 30–31, 60, 76, 77
Imrie, John, 201n1
Ince, Onur Ulas, 1
Indigenous peoples, 4, 14, 38, 94, 111, 124, 189; in *Carpentaria*, 18–19, 115, 204n7; dispossession of lands, 1, 3, 62, 159, 163, 184–85; existing on margins of the state, 33, 91–92; healing forms regarded as inferior to Western medicine, 58, 60, 76–80, 187; labor of, 15, 16, 19, 186; regarded as lazy, 14, 16, 26; sovereignty of, 168, 190, 191. *See also* Aboriginal peoples; *and individual groups of Indigenous peoples*
infant rape, 133, 135–37, 150, 202n8. *See also* child rape; children, sexual assault of; rape; sexual assault
instrumentalization, 5, 139, 165; of Aboriginal bodies, 169, 181, 204n7; capitalist, 100, 168; of human beings, 54, 60, 172; logic of, 33, 107–8; of objects, 171; of Western medicine, 75–76; of white liberalism, 129
intersectionality, theory of, 128–29, 140
Intervention, the. *See* Northern Territory National Emergency Response (NTER, Australia)
interventions: effluent-enabling, 149–57;

exceeding resistance, 31; foreign, 79; humanitarian, 3, 58, 199n12; medical, 81; public health, 18, 167
isiZulu peoples, 84, 85; culture of, 41; language of, 155, 196n10, 201n1

Jackson, Zakiyyah Iman, 28, 29, 34, 196n9
Jamaica, 66, 68, 199n10. *See also* Maroons
Jolly, Rosemary J., 195n1

Kaplan, Arthur, 52
Kappelman, Ben Desmond, 201n2
Kasdorf, Julia, 124
Katz, Louis, 200n15
Kim, Claire Jean, 25–26, 39
Kimmerer, Robin Wall, *Braiding Sweetgrass*, 38
Kinshasa (Republic of Congo): origins of HIV in, 19–20. *See also* Leopoldville (Republic of Congo)
Kirk, Robert, 52
Kłodziński, Stanisław, 74
Krog, Antjie, 137
KwaZulu-Natal (KZN, South Africa): gender-based violence in, 140–41, 155; HIV/AIDS epidemic in, 14, 41, 54, 134–35, 137, 140, 141; youth sexual relationships, 201n1

labor, 15, 87, 177; Aboriginal, 160, 165, 169, 175, 176; exploitative practices of, 3, 26, 57–58, 64, 68, 74–75, 84, 124, 169, 204n3; indentured, 20, 51, 136, 159; of Indigenous peoples, 15, 16, 19, 186. *See also* slavery/slaves
LaCapra, Dominick, 139–40, 141, 143
Land, Isaac, 64, 65, 67
language. *See* English (language); isiZulu peoples, language of

Lansing, Robert, 69
late capitalism, 18, 61, 166, 177–78, 180. *See also* capitalism; colonial capitalism; global capitalism; settler capitalism
late liberalism, 144, 146–49, 176, 191–92. *See also* liberalism; neoliberalism
Laub, Dori, 13
Lazarus, Neil, 29–30, 195n2
Leavis, F. R.: "Great Tradition" proposed by, 89–90
Lemey, Phillipe, 80
Leopoldville (Republic of Congo), 19–20, 52
Lesotho: HIV/AIDS in, 77–79, 80
Lethabo King, Tiffany, 4
let live, make die, 73–75. *See also* biopolitics; make die
Levi, Primo, 151
Lewis, Stephen, 197n20
liberal capitalism, 168, 169
liberalism, 129. *See also* late liberalism; neoliberalism; settler liberalism
Liberia: Ebola epidemic in, 53, 54, 81; history of, 66, 67–69, 73
Limbaugh, Rush, 53, 55
Little Children Are Sacred report (LCASR), 162, 163, 166
living, the: relations with the unborn and the ancestors, 35–37, 39, 57, 186, 189
Lukács, Georg, *The Meaning of Contemporary Realism*, 30

Macoun, Alissa, 163
make die, 84, 180. *See also* let live, make die
manngyin, Yarralin, 170–71, 173, 187
maroons, 66–67, 68, 199n10. *See also* Jamaica

materialism. *See* animism, materialist; new materialism
Mbembe, Achille, 54, 74–75, 84
McClure, Kristie, 180
McKegney, Sam, 27
medicine: postcolonial, 59–62, 76; precolonial, 59–60; privatization of, 85–86; rescue, 76–80; tropical, 187; Western regarded as superior to Indigenous, 58, 60, 76–80, 187. *See also* disease(s); health/health care
Mende peoples, 65–66
MERS (Middle East respiratory syndrome), 21
Million, Dian, 124, 156, 190–91, 201n6
MINUSTAH, 72–73
modernism: genres of, 150
modernity, 24, 82–83, 99; capitalist, 26, 38
Morton, Timothy. *See* hyperobjectivity/hyperobjects, Morton's concept of
mousetrap, 87–90, 94; in *Heat and Light*, 112; in *The Reactive*, 108
Mphahlele, Es'kia, 196n8; *And the Birds Flew Away* (proposed novel), 28, 38, 197n16; on burial of afterbirth, 37, 39; narrative by, 46. *See also* humanism, African, Mphahlele's concept of
Musselman, 75, 85; as racialized term, 74, 199n13

narratives, 17, 24, 28, 46, 138–42, 164, 187. *See also* bildungsroman; novels
nation-state: in *Carpentaria*, 160, 179; formation of, 61, 63–75; power of, 54; treatment of minorities, 191; violence inflicted by, 32, 90, 115. *See also* governance; state, the
Native peoples. *See* Aboriginal peoples; Indigenous peoples; and *individual groups of Indigenous peoples*
necropolitics, 75. *See also* politics; thanatopolitics
Neocleous, Mark, 195n4, 204n7
neocolonialism, 29, 31, 58, 85, 149, 159. *See also* colonialism; postcolonialism; settler colonialism
neoliberalism, 30–31, 129–30, 192, 195n4, 204n7. *See also* late liberalism; settler liberalism
new materialism, 27–28, 37, 195n1
Nietzsche, Friedrich Wilhelm, 82
Nixon, Rob, 142
Nolen, Stephanie, 46
nonhuman animals, 6, 21, 35, 44; companion, 51, 62; otherness of, 25, 159
normate, the, 129, 153, 189; behavior change interventions, 154–55; genre of man and, 126–27, 184, 186; genre of the human and, 130, 191; of liberal humanism, 159–60; sexual assault concept of, 126–28
Northern Territory National Emergency Response (NTER, Australia), 3, 132, 161–63, 166, 181
novels, 25, 176, 181–82. *See also* bildungsroman; narratives
Ntshanga, Masande, *The Reactive*, 87, 94–121; effluence in, 85–86, 90, 93; *Heat and Light* compared to, 87, 89–90, 186–88; resilience in, 100, 108

Obama, Barack, 52–53, 54
object(s), 25–26, 62, 143, 171, 187, 195n1. *See also* hyperobjectivity/hyperobjects, Morton's concept of
Oliver, Kelly, 12, 13, 14, 92, 126, 151, 152, 153, 160, 161
oppression: histories of, 142, 150; systemic, 128, 137–38

otherness/others, 37, 83, 123, 187; affirmation of, 92–93; colonialist-capitalist, 74, 75, 90–91, 188; cultural setting of, 77, 189; nonhuman, 25, 159; politics of, 198n6; suffering of, 147, 148–49

pandemics, 17–18, 19. *See also* Covid-19
Parry, Benita, 195n2
patriarchy, 131, 144–47, 161, 166, 180
Pennsylvania, 87, 89, 94, 98–99. *See also* Three Mile Island leak
Pennsylvania State University. *See* Sandusky, Gerry, sexual assault scandal
persistence, 4, 31, 36, 126, 169, 190, 201n6; depicted in *Carpentaria*, 175–77; of effluent communities, 86, 93, 153; under global capitalism, 112–21; harm reduction as, 163–66; use of term, 195n4
Philip, Marlene NourbeSe, 27; *Zong!*, 6, 8–12. *See also* Zong (slave ship)
Pierre, Joseph M., 203n11
Piot, Peter, 79
placenta: use of term, 196n13. *See also* afterbirth
politics: of affect, 144; of body-snatching, 11, 12; of colonialism, 57; of decolonialism, 166; of the effluent, 7; of immunity, 83, 84, 85, 112–13; of intentionality, 61; marginal, 54; of neocolonialism, 85; of otherness, 198n6; racial, 55, 82–83; of recognition, 12–13, 92, 143, 160, 161, 182; of self, 93; of sympathy, 148–49; textual, 29. *See also* biopolitics; necropolitics; thanatopolitics
postcolonialism, 1, 165; communities under, 23–24, 91–92, 99–100; exotic of, 170–71, 187; illness and debility in, 73–75, 83; inadequacy to the effluent, 29–47; medical education and, 75, 77; pathological, 29–32
post-Enlightenment, 2, 16, 24, 25, 27, 35–36. *See also* Enlightenment
posthumanism, 1, 24, 27–28, 37, 196n9, 204n3
postmodernism, 30, 150
poststructuralism, 29–31
Povinelli, Elizabeth, 27, 143, 147, 159, 160, 169, 174–76, 177, 179–80, 181
power: anthropocentric, 198n8; colonial, 30–31, 38; geontological, 176, 177; to let live, make die, 73–75; to make die, 180, 184; sovereign, 54, 74, 84; utopian will to, 61; white male heteronormative, 124
precarity: Butler's concept of, 4, 32–33, 90–93
prejudice. *See* racism
Preston, Richard, *The Hot Zone*, 80
Preston-Whyte, Eleanor, 20
Puar, Jasbir, 73, 75, 83
public health, 13–14, 20, 63, 136, 159. *See also* fifth-wave public-health theory; health/health care
Pybus, Oliver, 20, 79, 80

race, 17, 25, 26, 75
racism, 55, 65, 70, 136, 196n9; grievance under, 57, 189; Hegelian, 40, 197n18. *See also* apartheid; Black Lives Matter
rape, 126, 127, 129, 145, 171, 194–95n10; trauma of, 139, 141, 148; on U.S. college campuses, 127, 132, 145–46; victim-survivors of, 137–38, 151. *See also* child rape; gender-based-violence (GBV); infant rape; sexual assault
Rastafarianism, 68

rationality: Enlightenment culture of, 28, 34
Ravenscroft, Alison, 170, 173, 176, 178, 187
realism, 94–95, 171
recognition. *See* politics, of recognition
reservoir species, 20–21, 200n15
resilience, 27, 34, 78, 95, 177, 188; of child-rape survivors, 134, 140; of colonial capitalism, 27; communal, 135, 144; effluent, 112–21; in face of structural violence, 156–57; of global capitalism, 84; medical concept of, 166–67; as neoliberal tool, 195n4, 204n7; in reaction to trauma, 143; in *The Reactive*, 100, 108
resistance, 24, 31, 86, 195n3
Richardson, Samuel, 89–90
Rifkin, Mark, 27, 204n6
rights, 126, 159–60, 190. *See also* human right-making; human rightness; human rights; human rights violations (HRVs)
rituals, 36–37, 39, 176, 189
Rose, Deborah Bird, 170
Ross, Fiona, 137
Rothberg, Michael, 149
Rouse, Joseph, 196n9
Rushdie, Salman, *Midnight's Children*, 195n2
Ryn, Zdzisław, 74

Sabsay, Leticia, 195n3
Sanders, Bernie: campaign for the presidency, 32
Sandusky, Gerry, sexual assault scandal, 127–28, 142
SARS-CoV, 20–22. *See also* Covid-19
savior mentality, 62, 110, 126, 132
Schmaljohn, Alan, 200n15
Schmidt, Hans, 70

Schocket, Andrew, 64, 65, 67
self-harm, 166–67, 168. *See also* addiction; HIV/AIDS, self-infecting; substance abuse
Seligman, Herbert J., 71–72
Senauth, Frank, 71
settler capitalism, 3, 75, 112, 126, 190. *See also* capitalism; colonial capitalism; global capitalism; late capitalism
settler-colonial capitalism, 16, 126, 138, 175–76
settler colonialism, 14, 17, 59, 61, 111, 124, 184, 189, 191; structural violence of, 125, 129–30, 138. *See also* colonialism; neocolonialism; postcolonialism
settler liberalism, 176. *See also* late liberalism; neoliberalism
sexual assault: causes of, 190; commodification's relation to, 171; global context, 123–57; intergenerational perpetration, 131, 136; male-on-male, 132–33; in the military, 201n2; perpetrators of, 126–29, 131–32, 146–51, 153; perpetrator-victims of, 125, 128, 142, 149; prevention and healing, 149–57; in South Africa, 127, 134–36; trauma of, 126, 138–42, 148, 150–51; victim-survivors of, 13, 124–28, 131–32, 134–35, 137–38, 142, 150–51, 153–55, 191, 201n2. *See also* child rape; children, sexual assault of; gender-based-violence (GBV); infant rape; rape; women, sexual assault of
shame: in *Heat and Light*, 103–5, 116–17; sexual assault victims' feelings of, 151–53
Sharpe, Christina, 4
Sherbro peoples, 64
Shoah. *See* Holocaust

Sierra Leone: history of, 64–67, 69, 73
simultaneous reading, 183–92
Slaughter, Joseph, 27, 166; on bildungsroman, 24, 26, 90, 93, 164; *Human Rights, Inc.*, 25; on *Nervous Conditions*, 96
slavery/slaves, 1, 4, 60, 136, 159, 167; colonial capitalism's dependence on, 51, 57, 68, 74, 75, 84; historical figures of, 56–57; rebellion against, 69–71; reparations for, 73, 84; settling freed slaves in African colonies and Haiti, 63–73; as structural violence, 125; subventions from, 13, 26; trauma of, 139–40; U.S. role in, 53, 54. See also body-snatching; commodification/commodities; labor, exploitative practices of; Philip, Marlene NourbeSe, *Zong!*; *Zong* (slave ship)
slow becoming, 183–92
slow death, 73, 75, 117, 169, 189–90
social and economic determinants of health (SEDH), 59, 61, 198n3
South Africa: Blacks in, 14, 115; extractive industries in, 100–101; HIV/AIDS epidemic in, 14, 24, 39–47, 54–55, 78, 110, 115, 127, 134–37, 140–41, 154, 197n20, 201n1; sexual abuse in, 127, 134–36. See also apartheid; KwaZulu-Natal (KZN, South Africa); Lesotho; Soweto township (Johannesburg, South Africa)
sovereignty, 12, 61, 63, 74–75, 84; of Indigenous peoples, 168, 190, 191; power of, 54, 74, 84; state, 5, 11–12, 84
Soweto township (Johannesburg, South Africa), 13, 197n17
Soyinka, Wole, 27, 36, 39; *Death and the King's Horseman*, 186

speakability: Butler's concept of, 6–7, 10, 11, 152, 153, 167; of capitalism's failures, 87. See also unspeakability
spectator-reader privilege, 142–49
Stankiewicz, Ignatius, 43, 44. See also Centocow mission
state, the, 3, 23, 55, 60, 161, 190; colonialist-capitalist, 57, 91–92, 188; debility in, 50–51; neoliberal, 31, 192; postcolonial, 35, 79; role in right to health care, 24, 44, 49, 54, 110, 118; settler, 57, 64; sovereignty of, 5, 11–12, 84; as subject, 185–86. See also governance; nation-state; violence, state-inflicted
statelessness, 2, 195–96n7
Stronger Futures Act (Australia), 162–63
structural violence, 2, 12, 55, 57, 124, 143, 194n5; of colonial capitalism, 51, 58, 63, 86, 115, 166, 191; effects on health, 59, 85, 198n7; Galtung's definition of, 128–29; of global capitalism, 1, 18, 61; intersectional, 140, 141; overcoming, 189–90; recognition of, 29–30; resilience in face of, 156–57; of settler colonialism, 125, 129–30, 138; state-inflicted, 93, 161. See also gender-based-violence (GBV); rape; sexual assault; violence
subjectivities, 24, 85, 173; Aboriginal, 189; bourgeois, 31; in *Carpentaria*, 166; co-constituted, 153, 187, 189, 191, 193n3; effluent, 11–15, 35; environmental, 6, 174; forms of, 5–6, 118; human, 63; individual, 151; of matter, 196n9; of slow becoming, 191–92; sovereign, 12, 84; of the state, 185, 186; of victims, 126, 132
subjects, 12, 75, 110, 143; of bildungsroman, 92–93; co-constituted, 3,

36, 117, 120; colonial capitalist, 26, 64, 74; discrete, 7–8, 11; human, 3, 5, 24–28, 62, 186–87; myth of, 90–93; normative, 11, 13, 25; of property, 10–11; reactives/reactors, 95; rights-bearing/rights-seeking, 161, 163–66, 181–82; of trauma, 144, 153. *See also* citizen-subjects; effluent subjects

sub-Saharan Africa: animist traditions in, 34–36; Hegel on, 197n18; HIV/AIDS epidemic in, 39–40, 46, 51, 55; Indigenous peoples in, 16; postcolonies of, 73. *See also* Liberia; Sierra Leone; South Africa; West Africa

substance abuse, 166–67; colonial capitalism and, 87–121; harm reduction strategy applied to, 159; among Indigenous peoples, 18. *See also* addiction; self-harm

suffering, 40–47; Berlant's theory of, 125, 143–44; in *Carpentaria*, 171, 182; caused by disease, 53, 187; deep, 81; of others, 147, 148–49; recognizing, 11–12; spectators of, 127, 143–44

sustainability, 28, 79, 119, 165, 174, 180–81, 190–91

TallBear, Kim, 159
Tatem, Andrew J., 80
Temne peoples, 65–66
territorialism, 1, 159
thanatopolitics, 82–83. *See also* necropolitics; politics
Three Mile Island leak, 88–89, 102, 200n1
transmission species, 19–21
trauma, 165, 190, 191, 202–3n9; of apartheid, 136, 140, 141, 150; of colonization, 141, 191; as event, 134, 142–43, 150–51, 202n8; exceptionalism of, 123–57; gender-based, 136, 137–38; reactions to, 203n11, 203n12; of sexual assault, 126, 138–42, 148, 150–51; theories of, 4, 126, 138–42, 142–49

Trotsky, Leon: theory of combined but uneven development, 89
Trump, Donald J., 69, 145, 199n11, 203n13
Truth and Reconciliation Commission (TRC): in Canada, 190–91; in South Africa, 109, 137–38, 194n5

unborn, the: abortion issue and, 196n12; relations with the living and the ancestors, 35–37, 39, 57, 186, 189
ungrievability: Butler's concept of, 4, 12, 40, 90, 91, 147. *See also* grievability
United Nations, *Declaration on Human Rights* (UNDHR), 2, 3, 17; Aboriginal/Indigenous life excluded from, 160, 161; treatment of genre of the human, 51, 57, 63, 160
United Nations, *Declaration on the Rights of Indigenous Peoples* (UNDRIP), 160
United Nations High Commission on Human Rights (UNHCHR), 16
unspeakability, 24, 39, 47, 52, 151; Butler's concept of, 10–13; figures of, 6–7, 58. *See also* speakability
utopianism, 15, 57–58, 60, 61, 64, 83–86

Veracini, Lorenzo, 193n2
Verwoerd, Hendrik Frensch, 200n4
violence, 85, 124; colonialist-capitalist, 94, 112, 198n7; against HIV-positive people, 140–41; intergenerational, 136, 162; interpersonal, 140, 194n5; racialized, 85, 136; sexual, 131, 138, 146–47; state-inflicted, 13, 32–33, 90,

91, 115, 131, 134, 164. *See also* gender-based-violence (GBV); gross human rights violations (GHRVs); sexual assault; structural violence

Wacquant, L., 87
Wagner, Valeria, 95
waiting-with, practice of, 111, 118, 120
Waanyi, 178, 187. *See also* Wright, Alexis, *Carpentaria*
Warwick Research Collective (WReC): combined and uneven development theory, 89–90, 95
waste: from effluent bodies, 5, 7, 14, 39, 46; lead, 89, 174
Watt, Ian: history of the novel, 89–90
Weheliye, Alexander G., 12, 74, 125, 131, 199n13
West Africa, 51–52, 85. *See also* Liberia; Sierra Leone
whiteness/whites, 36, 39, 62, 75, 129, 182, 185; belief in their superiority to Blacks, 55, 64, 68, 69; colonization practices, 3, 94, 171; right to health care, 88; savior mentality, 62, 110, 126, 132. *See also* savior mentality
Wild, Rex, 162, 163
Winston, Jameis, 147, 156
Winter, Yves, 129
women: Black, 17, 55; perceived vulnerability of, 131, 132; sexual assault of, 124, 126–27, 135–38, 141, 145. *See also* gender-based-violence (GBV)
World Health Organization (WHO): constitution, 15; definition of SDEH, 198n3; response to SARS-CoV, 20; on right to health and health care, 49–50

Wright, Alexis, 130, 190; *Grog War*, 168
Wright, Alexis, *Carpentaria*, 159–82, 186–87; anthropocentric values posed by, 169–73; effluent subjects in, 157; genre of the human in, 166, 188; harm reduction strategy in, 188; Indigenous peoples in, 18–19, 115, 204n7; nation-state in, 160, 179; as normative human-rights narrative, 181; persistence depicted in, 175–76; suffering in, 171, 182; timescape in, 169–73; youths in, 189. *See also Waanyi*
Wynter, Sylvia, 2, 23, 123. *See also* genre of man, Wynter's concept of; genre of the human, Wynter's concept of

Yeats, W. B., 57; "Crazy Jane Talks with the Bishop," 6–8, 10

Žižek, Slavoj, 95
zoe, 74; *bios* versus, 75, 83
zombies, 56–57, 58, 70; as revenants, 80–86
Zong (slave ship), 13, 14, 15. *See also* Philip, Marlene NourbeSe, *Zong!*
zooanthroponoses, 22
zoonoses, 51; use of term, 22
zorg. *See* health/health care

ROSEMARY J. JOLLY is Sparks Chair of Literature and Human Rights at the Pennsylvania State University. She is author of *Colonization, Violence, and Narration* and *Cultured Violence: Narrative, Social Suffering, and Engendering Human Rights in Contemporary South Africa* and coeditor of *Writing South Africa*.